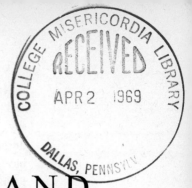
WATER AND ELECTROLYTES

Implications for Nursing Practice

ISABEL E. DUTCHER, M.A., R.N.

Assistant Professor, Medical-Surgical Nursing
Rutgers University
Newark, New Jersey

SANDRA B. FIELO, M.A., R.N.

Instructor in Nursing
Middlesex County College
Edison, New Jersey

THE MACMILLAN COMPANY · *New York*
COLLIER-MACMILLAN LIMITED · *London*

... In what manner the sea produced the mysterious and wonderful stuff called protoplasm we cannot say. In its warm, dimly lit waters the unknown conditions of temperature, pressure and saltiness must have been the critical ones for the creation of life from non-life. At any rate, they produced the result that neither the alchemists with their crucibles nor modern scientists in their laboratories have been able to achieve.

RACHEL CARSON,
The Sea Around Us

Library of Congress catalog card number: 67–13638

THE MACMILLAN COMPANY, New York
COLLIER-MACMILLAN CANADA, LTD., Toronto, Ontario

PRINTED IN THE UNITED STATES OF AMERICA

FOREWORD

DURING the past several decades the nursing profession has outgrown its primary role of the rote executing of physicians' orders. More and more its members have been studying the underlying bases for diagnosis and therapy. Certainly this is all to the good. It can result only in the increasing significance of the nurses' role on the health team. Even more important, it will contribute to better patient care.

Perhaps in no medical area does the nurses' new role have greater meaning than in the field of body fluid disturbances. Why should this be so? Body fluid disturbances represent acute ailments that can change for the worse in hours or even minutes. The patient with such a disturbance requires constant observation, and it is the nursing staff, not the physician, who observes the patient 24 hours a day, albeit through three shifts.

The nurse responsible for the patient with a body fluid disturbance must not only closely observe him—she must also report new developments promptly to the physician, regulate the administration of parenteral fluids, see that orders for oral fluids are carried out, and employ judgment in executing the physicians' orders, not hesitating to recommend deviations from the orders in case of need. Finally, she performs the invaluable role of supervising the measuring and recording of intake and output.

How important are body fluid disturbances? They are vastly important. Any patient is a candidate for one of them. Frequently the body fluid disturbance induced by a disease assumes greater importance than the primary ailment. Diarrhea is a case in point. The development of potent new pharmaceutical agents has increased, rather than decreased, the incidence of fluid imbalances. As an example, some 11 different types of medical therapy, and at least five categories of surgical therapy, frequently induce a potassium deficit. As Dr. J. L. B. Montenegro, of São Paulo, Brazil, has perceptively stated: "Body fluid disturbances represent the common denominator of a host of illnesses."

Despite the burgeoning significance of body fluid disturbances and of the nurses' role in their management, the number of thoughtful nursing textbooks on the subject has been small indeed. The authors, having repeatedly been forced to search out needed nursing information in widely dispersed sources that were either too simple or too complex, decided to write a text supplement that would present the middle ground of sophisticated but understandable information related to fluid imbalances.

The book is primarily aimed at the professional nurse, especially the serious student, and the nursing instructor. Most helpful in accomplishing the goal is the inclusion of a patient care study for each of the major imbalance categories, including the plan of care from the nursing standpoint. The book encourages the nurse to have sufficient knowledge and understanding so that she can make valid and pertinent observations—then know what to do about them.

It is good we have this book. It has been badly needed for a long time.

W. D. SNIVELY, JR., M.D.
Clinical Professor, Department of Pediatrics
Medical College of Alabama

PREFACE

IN THE seventeenth century, Thomas Latta experimented with the use of salt water as an intravenous replacement solution; however, the more sophisticated use of water and electrolytes for parenteral replacement is of fairly recent origin. The rationale underlying this therapy is the maintenance of a tenable level of homeostasis enabling patients to survive illness. All illnesses cause some degree of water and electrolyte imbalance.

The problem of water and electrolyte imbalance is extremely complex and not completely understood by any one person; yet knowledge available is prerequisite to the understanding of what is happening to a patient during illness. Although it is within the province of the physician to prescribe the kinds and amounts of replacement solution, it is within the province of the nurse to make pertinent observations concerning the efficacy of the ongoing therapy. To do this, she must have certain information.

The purpose of this book is to provide nurses with pertinent information related to these balances and imbalances in water and electrolytes. The material relative to this problem is voluminous, complex, and disseminated in a multitude of sources. We have attempted to compile the information that a nurse needs to have available in order to understand, to observe, and to interpret competently those problems related to water and electrolyte balance.

The material is presented in three sections: equilibrium of water and electrolytes (the normal), disequilibrium of water and electrolytes (the imbalance), and replacement therapy. We have attempted to stress particular implications for nurses by using actual patient care studies.

It is our hope that nurses will develop an appreciation for the intricate, awesome beauty that nature has bestowed upon us in the dynamic equilibrium of water and electrolytes in the body.

I. E. D.
S. B. F.

v

ACKNOWLEDGMENTS

THE authors are indebted to the many persons who encouraged them during the preparation of this manuscript. Without a doubt, our students should be the first to be acknowledged, for it is they who raised the questions and sought the answers that led the authors to the preparation of a text supplement that would not only help them to find some of the answers, but also stimulate them to raise more questions.

Grateful appreciation is due William D. Snively, Jr., M.D., Clinical Professor of Pediatrics, Medical College of Alabama, and Vice President of Medical Affairs, Mead Johnson Co., for his encouragement, critical review of the manuscript, and valuable suggestions.

Words of appreciation are also due:

L. Bernice Chapman, Dean, College of Nursing, Rutgers, The State University of New Jersey, and Mrs. Rose Channing, Chairman, Department of Nurse Education, Middlesex County College, Edison, New Jersey, for their counsel and support.

Miss Carol Belardo, senior nursing student at Rutgers, The State University of New Jersey, for typing the manuscript.

Mrs. Alice I. Bernstein, medical staff librarian, Perth Amboy General Hospital, for her generous help in searching out references.

Mr. Henry Van Swearingen, editor in the College and Professional Division of The Macmillan Company, for his help and guidance in the preparation of the book for publication.

And finally, but by no means least, two very patient and understanding husbands, James and Joel.

I. E. D.
S. B. F.

CONTENTS

SECTION I
The State of Equilibrium

CHAPTER 1

The Fluid Matrix of the Body

LIKE the intricate mechanism of a complex piece of machinery or the marvelous blending of a magnificent painting, equilibrium within the body is a superb blending of continuous, dynamic, and ever-functioning processes aimed at maintaining a life-sustaining balance. Let one of the numerous homeostatic regulators fail in its precise job, and the balance is disturbed.

The body fluids carry on their dynamic function within two major fluid compartments—the cell fluid, or intracellular, and the tissue (interstitial) fluid and plasma (intravascular) fluid, or extracellular. The extracellular fluid comprises the environment for all cells. It is composed chiefly of water and inorganic salts. Intracellular fluid is more complex and, in addition to water and inorganic salts, contains the organic constituents of protoplasm.

Equilibrium of the fluids and electrolytes is maintained within a very narrow range of normal values by numerous homeostatic mechanisms. In illness this equilibrium is upset. When this occurs, physiological mechanisms operate to re-establish the premorbid level. The object of therapy, therefore, is to help the ill person to regain and to maintain the balance that is a requisite of health.

Some Basic Chemical Facts That Relate to Body Water and Electrolytes

IONS

Ions are atoms, or groups of atoms, carrying an electric charge due to the loss or gain of electrons from particles that were previously electrically neutral. When electrons are lost, a net positive charge is left on the particle; such a charged particle is a cation. When electrons

3

are gained, with a resulting excess of electrons, the particle carries a negative charge; the negatively charged particle is an anion. The terms "cation" and "anion" are derived from the positive and negative poles of a battery. In solution, the positively charged ions are attracted to the negative pole, or cathode. The negatively charged ions are attracted to the positively charged pole, or anode.

Gain or loss of a single electron results in a univalent ion. Ions with a gain or loss of two and three electrons are divalent and trivalent ions. In solution, ions of like charge cannot exist alone; they must be balanced by an equal number of oppositely charged ions. In solution each ion exists as an independent particle, but the solution as a whole is electrically neutral.

IONIZATION

When sodium chloride, for example, goes into solution, the salt dissociates into its ionic constituents, the sodium ion and the chloride ion:

$$NaCl \rightarrow Na^+ + Cl^-$$

The two dissociated ions are relatively independent of each other, existing in the solution as independent entities. The term "ionization" means that the sodium chloride exists in solution in ionic rather than molecular form.

Substances capable of dissociating into ions when in solution are called electrolytes. Substances that do not ionize in solution and thus do not carry an electrical charge because they have no group in their molecules that can dissociate are called nonelectrolytes. Glucose, for example, is a nonelectrolyte, because it exists in solution as a nondissociated, electrically neutral glucose molecule.

Compounds that ionize completely in solution are referred to as strong electrolytes. Generally, these comprise the inorganic acids, bases, and most of the soluble inorganic salts. Compounds that ionize in solution to a limited degree are referred to as weak electrolytes and comprise most organic acids and bases.

BODY WATER

Physiochemical activities of life take place in solution in which water is the solvent. Water is the largest single constituent of all living organisms. The proper functioning of any cell depends on the correct concentration and unimpeded movement of water between the various water compartments, viz, intravascular, interstitial, and intracellular. As a solvent, water is ideal, because more substances dissolve to an appreciable extent in water than in any other liquid. Owing to the great solvent power of water it does not exist in the body, or, in fact, in any place in nature, as pure water but rather as a solution of salts and other molecular dispersions. The body liquids perform two vital services: (1) transportation of nutrient materials to and waste products from cells; (2) maintenance of physical-chemical constancy, in both intracellular and extracellular fluids.

PHYSICAL PROPERTIES OF WATER

In addition to the property of solvency, water possesses other physical properties to render it the ideal physiological solvent.

High Specific Heat of Water. The heat capacity of different materials is their specific heat—the specific heat of 1 gm of material at 1°C temperature is the number of calories (small) of heat that 1 gm of the material must collect to raise its temperature through 1°C. Water has a high specific heat, meaning that water collects more heat than other materials to result in the same temperature change. This high heat capacity of water is of vital significance. Because of this property the water component of blood is able to collect the considerable quantity of heat produced by cellular activity and carry it to the body surface, with less of a rise in temperature than would be the case if any other liquid were the heat-transporting medium.

High Latent Heat of Vaporization. This is a definite heat quantity for each substance and is the temperature at which the particular substance vaporizes. Latent heat of vaporization of a substance is the number of calories (small) of heat that 1 gm of the substance must absorb in order to change from the liquid to the gaseous state without undergoing any temperature change. The latent heat of vaporization of water is very high. From 2500 to 3500 calories (large) of heat per day is made in cells for living needs. This heat is carried by blood to the skin and lungs. The larger portion of this heat is used for vaporizing the water that is excreted at these areas, and since it is latent, this heat causes no increase in temperature. A small portion of the heat brought to body surfaces is radiated as appreciable heat which keeps the body warm and warms the surrounding air. The high latent heat of vaporization of water provides the major mechanism for body temperature control.

DISTRIBUTION OF BODY WATER

In the true physiological state, the water contained within the body does not recognize anatomical limits. The compartmentalization of water into the various water phases of the body is for the convenience of the physiologist.

In the adult human approximately 60 per cent of the total body weight is water; this proportion decreases with age. In the human neonate 77 per cent of total body weight is water, a percentage that falls sharply after birth to about four years of age and then levels off to a relatively constant level.[1] Total body water content is divided into two major compartments: the intracellular and the extracellular. The latter compartment is comprised of the intravascular and interstitial fluids. The distribution of water within these compartments is a dynamic constant. The compartmentalization of water in a lean adult is approximately:

1. Intracellular—40 per cent. A higher percentage of this is in the liver, striated muscles, and skin and a lower percentage in cartilage and bone.
2. Extracellular—20 per cent. 15 per cent of this is interstitial fluid and 5 per cent plasma.

Adipose tissue is relatively free of water; therefore, the percentage of body weight that is water is less in an obese than in a lean person. This deceptive appearance of an obese individual may lead the observer to overlook a state of dehydration.

Intracellular fluids consist of water and the cellular solutes and represent the site of cellular metabolic processes. Interstitial fluid lies outside cells and constitutes the aqueous cellular environment. It maintains a relatively constant environment within which normal cellular function can occur. This fluid is the pathway between cells and the intravascular fluid and allows for exchanges of material with the external environment.

Fluids located within such sites as the ducts of glands, the gastrointestinal tract, and the urinary collecting system are referred to as transcellular fluids.

INTERNAL TRANSFER OF FLUIDS

Water moves freely from one compartment to another because most living membranes permit the passage of water; that is, they are freely permeable to water molecules. It is the behavior of the solutes in a solution that influences the movement of water. The processes that allow for movement of water within and between the compartments are diffusion, osmosis, and active transport.

DIFFUSION

Diffusion of molecules according to a difference in concentration is the simplest type of fluid movement. In this type of transfer solutes and solvent diffuse from the area of their highest concentration in the direction of their least concentration until equilibrium is established.

OSMOSIS

Forces that are engendered by the process of osmosis are of the utmost importance in regulating the distribution of body water. Although the compositions of the intracellular and extracellular liquids differ considerably, the total concentration of solutes in each is about equal. This is because the cell membrane that separates the liquids is freely permeable to water.

In a true solution, molecules of water and molecules of solute are in continual random movement except when the temperature is at absolute zero ($-273°C$). As a result these molecules are continuously hitting against each other or any object in their way and rebounding. As a result of these constant random movements and the consequent rebounding, a pressure is established, called osmotic pressure. This pressure is proportional to the number of the dispersed solute particles. The higher the concentration of the solute particles, the greater the number of impacts between molecules, hence the greater the osmotic pressure of the solution. Conversely, the lesser the concentration of solute particles and the consequently reduced number of molecular impacts, the lower the osmotic pressure of the solution.

An important physiological phenomenon resulting from osmotic pressure is osmosis, which is the passage of molecules of water or of water and solute through a semipermeable membrane separating two solutions. A semipermeable membrane is one that is freely permeable to water but relatively impermeable to solute particles. Water will move across the membrane from a solution with a lesser concentration of particles into one with a higher concentration of particles; i.e., "water goes where the salt is."

The most important forces that tend to pull water into, or to prevent the escape of water from, the intracellular and extracellular compartments are the osmotic pressures exerted by the dissociated electrolytes in these compartments. In extracellular fluid the principal osmotic effects are exerted by sodium and chloride ions. In the intracellular fluid these effects are exerted by potassium, magnesium, phosphates, and proteinates. When the concentration of ions on either side of a membrane is altered, water moves quickly to re-establish osmotic equilibrium.

COLLOID OSMOTIC PRESSURE

Colloid osmotic pressure (oncotic) is the osmotic pressure that results from dispersed colloid particles. The largest group of these dispersed colloid particles in the body is protein. Albumins and globulins comprise most of the proteins of plasma. The relative concentration of these proteins in plasma is of great physiological importance. They are important because under normal conditions the colloidal osmotic pressure exerted almost entirely by the plasma proteins is the force that counterbalances the blood hydrostatic pressure at the arterial end of the blood capillaries. Electrolytes and water are freely diffusible across the capillary membrane; hence the osmotic pressure they exert is equal on both sides of the membrane. The capillary membrane is normally impermeable to the large protein molecules in blood, and their concentration is, therefore, greater within the blood capillaries. The osmotic pressure they exert is the pressure that pulls water back into the vascular system at the venous end of the capillaries, and this factor is of great significance in the maintenance of blood volume.*

The net effective pressure of the plasma proteins is 18 mm Hg.

The hydrostatic pressure inside the capillaries at the arterial end is about 32 mm Hg pressure; this falls to about 12 mm Hg at the venous end. (See Fig. 1.)

At the arterial end of the capillary the blood hydrostatic pressure exceeds the colloidal osmotic pressure of the plasma proteins, and water and dissolved particles are forced out of the vessel into the interstitial space. At the venous end the reverse situation occurs, and fluid is drawn back into the vessel. Filtration is fostered at the arterial

---

* The blood hydrostatic pressure forces water and solutes out into the tissue spaces at the arteriolar end of the capillaries, and the colloidal osmotic pressure is the force that pulls water and solutes from the tissue into blood at the venular end of the capillaries.

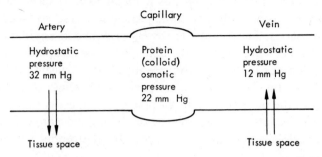

FIG. 1. Pressure differences within the capillary tend to push fluid into the tissue spaces at the arteriolar end of the capillary and pull fluid back into the capillary at its venular end.

end and reabsorption at the venous end. This small, but important, pressure effect of the plasma proteins is a major factor in maintaining an adequate blood volume.

ACTIVE TRANSPORT

Movement of fluid according to the laws of osmosis and diffusion does not sufficiently explain the movement of the solute ions. Ions possess the ability to penetrate cell membranes against a concentration gradient. This ability implies that the net movement of ions requires the expenditure of metabolically derived energy to effect the movement. The term "active transport" has been applied to any movement of solutes where there is an expenditure of energy to accomplish the movement.[2]

Active transport of solutes appears to be linked with special anatomical and spatial characteristics of membranes, specific enzyme systems, and the optimal concentration of ions. The cell membrane is a complex system that controls the movement of ions and metabolites in an active fashion. The exact mechanism underlying transfer by active transport is as yet unknown, although several attractive theories have been postulated. Active transport has been defined by Ussing, who states, ". . . we shall only speak of active transport where work has to be done to transfer ions across the membrane, whether this work is used to overcome a potential difference, a concentration difference or both."[3]

LYMPHATICS

The interstitial fluid is an ultrafiltrate of plasma. Therefore, it closely resembles plasma in its composition. The chief difference is this: interstitial fluid normally has a much lower concentration of protein than plasma, although some protein does escape through the blood capillaries. The lymphatic vessels originate as capillaries with blind ends. They are more permeable than blood capillaries. These vessels are unique in that they represent the only efficient mechanism for returning the large molecules, such as proteins, to the blood stream from the interstitial fluid and the gastrointestinal tract. These large molecules, after having entered the lymphatics, are transported from the periphery centrally and empty into the venous system.[4]

INTAKE AND OUTPUT OF WATER

With marked precision, the body normally maintains a balance between intake and water loss. During growth or a period of convalescence from illness, when new tissue is being formed or tissue is undergoing repair, water is retained. In these instances the output of water is less than the intake. This is because a large volume of water is bound to the protein of the newly formed tissue. The daily net turnover of water ranges from 3 to 6 per cent of the total body water. Balance is maintained if the water intake meets the two basic needs of causing loss of body heat by vaporization through lungs and skin and excreting solutes via the kidney. In addition, any abnormal loss of water from other routes must be regulated. For example, if a large volume of water is lost through the gastrointestinal tract, as in diarrhea or vomiting, less water is excreted by the kidneys and skin.

SOURCES OF WATER

The body has three major sources of water: (1) oral liquids, (2) water content of foods, and (3) water of oxidation. The largest fraction of daily intake is the water taken as beverages. However, solid foods have a high water content. Lean meat, for example, is about 75 per cent of water content by weight. Water is continually made available through the oxidation of foods, especially fats. An ordinary mixed diet will yield from 300 to 350 gm of water from the oxidation of foods. This yield is:

100 gm fat	107 gm water
100 gm carbohydrate	55 gm water
100 gm protein	41 gm water

AVENUES OF LOSS

Water is lost from the body through four avenues of exit: (1) expired air, (2) skin, (3) urine, and (4) feces. The water lost by vaporization from the lung and skin surfaces and the water lost in feces are obligatory losses and go on even when environmental temperatures are low.

Average Water Intake (Adult Male, Moderate Activity)		*Average Water Output* (Average Room Temperature and Humidity)	
Beverages	1350 ml	Urine	1500 ml
Water content of food	1000 ml	Stool	150 ml
Water of oxidation	350 ml	Insensible	700 ml

WATER OF VAPORIZATION OR INSENSIBLE WATER LOSS

Water is continuously being lost with the expired air from lungs and by vaporization from the skin surface. Total insensible (meaning "not aware") water loss per day is 600 to 1000 ml in a resting, nonfebrile adult. This rate of loss is accelerated by an increased metabolic rate (fever, exercise, panic). The insensible loss constitutes a loss of water only, without solutes.[5] The water vapor that is continually lost through the lungs accounts for some 25 per cent of heat loss. This water loss continues unabated even in the event of severe water deprivation.

SENSIBLE WATER LOSS

Sensible water loss is that which can be seen and felt over and above insensible perspiration. It constitutes a method for increased heat loss when there is increased heat production (fever, exercise, panic, etc.) or environmental temperature and humidity are increased. It is a product of sweat gland activity and contains both water and solutes.[6] Sweat is hypotonic in relation to other body fluids; thus more water is lost than solute.

There is evidence that adrenocortical hormones act on the tubules of the sweat glands inhibiting the excretion, especially if sweating has been extensive and prolonged.[6]

WATER EXCHANGE IN THE GASTROINTESTINAL TRACT

Large amounts of extracellular fluid are transferred daily into the stomach and intestines. Gamble[7] has estimated an average daily loss of an average daily volume of 8200 ml, divided as follows:

Saliva	1500 ml
Gastric secretion	2500 ml
Bile	500 ml
Pancreatic juice	700 ml
Intestinal mucosa	3000 ml
	8200 ml

This fluid serves its function in digestion and absorption and then passes on into the ileum and proximal colon, where it is almost entirely reabsorbed, since feces normally contain only 100 to 150 ml of water. This volume of fluid is more than twice the volume of blood plasma (3500 ml); thus the loss of large amounts of fluid from the gastrointestinal tract can cause serious consequences to the patient.

THIRST

One of the essential factors in the regulation and maintenance of the balance between water intake and its output is thirst. The sensation of thirst is a subjective phenomenon and is a major factor determining fluid intake. The chief stimulus to this sensation depends not only on cellular hypohydration but also on an increase in the hypertonicity (increased osmotic forces) of the body fluids. (One way to illustrate this is to cite the increased need for water when you eat salted nuts, potato chips, pretzels, and the like.) Additional stimuli to thirst include decreased circulating blood volume during hemorrhage and shock, drying of the oral mucous membranes, individual habits, and emotional factors, such as fear and panic. These stimuli may be inadequate or absent in the sick individual and thus are not reliable as indicators of the individual's need for fluids. Clinically, it has been observed that the edematous patient may be thirsty and that dehydrated patients often are not. A thirst or drinking center probably exists in the hypothalamus, where the cells are hypersensitive to changes in the osmotic pressure of blood. Increased osmotic pressure of blood stimulates the sensation of thirst, and fluids are taken to restore the balance.

UNITS OF MEASUREMENT

Since the compounds and ions of extracellular water interact with one another as molecules and ions, it is best to express concentrations of the components in divisions permitting comparison of interrelations between them. Units of measurement for this purpose are mol (M), millimol (mM), milliequivalent (mEq), and milliosmol (mOsm).

Mol and Millimol. A mol of a substance is the molecular weight of that substance in grams. For example, the chemical formula for potassium hydroxide is KOH. The molecular weight is $39 + 16 + 1 = 56.0$ gm. One mol of potassium hydroxide equals 56 gm; 1 millimol of potassium hydroxide is 1/1000 of 56 gm, or 56 mg. Mol or millimol is applicable to any of the ions. One mol of any ion is the sum of the atomic weights expressed in grams, e.g.

1 mol Na^+	23.0 gm
1 mol K^+	39.1 gm
1 mol Ca^{++}	40.0 gm
1 mol Cl^-	35.5 gm
1 mol SO_4^{--}	96.0 gm
	(sum of atomic weights)

One millimol of any of these ions is 1/1000 of a mol.

Milliosmol. The unit of measurement of osmotic pressure is the osmol. If 1 molecular weight of an un-ionized substance is dissolved in a liter of water it exerts 1 osmol, or 1000 milliosmol, of pressure. However, if the substance is completely ionized (e.g., K^+ OH^-), then the solution that contains 1 molecular weight of substance actually contains twice as many osmotically active particles, and this solution is said to exert 2 osmols, or 2000 milliosmols, of osmotic pressure.

Equivalents and Milliequivalents. Electrolytes are of physiological importance because of the number of particles present per unit volume (mol or millimol) and because of the number of charges per unit valence (equivalent or milliequivalent).

Equivalent and milliequivalent are units of measurement referring to combining equivalents or chemical activity. An equivalent of an ion is the sum of its atomic weights divided by the valence. A milli-equivalent is 1/1000 of 1 equivalent. For example:

Na^+:

Atomic weight	valence	equivalent
23	$\div$ $+1$	$=$ $+23$

Ca^{++}:

Atomic weight	valence	equivalent
40	$\div$ $+2$	$=$ $+20$

Therefore, 23 gm Na^+ and 20 gm Ca^{++} are equivalent, or both quantities possess the same number of positive charges.

EXAMPLE

If there are 10 mg per 100 ml of Ca in a solution, the mEq value would be determined as follows:

$$mEq/L = \frac{mg\% \times 10 \times valence}{atomic\ weight}$$

$$\frac{10 \times 10 \times 2}{40} = 5\ mEq\ Ca\ in\ 1\ liter\ of\ solution$$
containing 10 mg/100 ml

When concentrations of each ionic constituent of extracellular water are expressed in terms of milliequivalents per liter, the sum of all the positively charged ions (cations) exactly equals the sum of all the negatively charged ions (anions). Thus every positively charged ion must be balanced by a negatively charged ion. Milliequivalent measurement indicates the chemical activity of a solution, rather than its weight.

KIDNEY AND HORMONAL CONTROL OF WATER METABOLISM

The kidneys are the principal ultimate regulators of the internal environment. By virtue of their function they are the chief organs of homeostasis. The main responsibility for regulation of water, electrolyte, and hydrogen ion devolves upon the kidneys.

The functional and anatomical unit of the kidney is the nephron. Each kidney is estimated to contain 1,000,000 of these units. A nephron is composed of two functionally distinct parts (1) the glomerulus, primarily a vascular structure, and (2) the uriniferous tubule. The glomerulus is a tuft of capillaries partly encapsulated within a double endothelial capsule. The tubule is lined by endothelial cells and consists of the proximal convoluted tubule, loop of Henle, and distal convoluted tubule. Each distal tubule empties into a collecting tubule.

The glomerulus acts as an ultrafilter and filters from blood a dilute, protein-free fluid. This act of ultrafiltration is mainly a physical process which is dependent on the blood pressure within the glomerulus. The glomerular blood pressure is some 60 to 70 per cent of the mean arterial pressure, or about 75 mm Hg pressure. The opposing force to this is the colloid osmotic pressure of the plasma proteins in the glomerular capillaries and the tension within the glomerular capsule. The protein osmotic pressure is about 25 mm, and the capsular pressure is 10 mm. Therefore, the net effective filtration pressure is 75 minus 35, or 40 mm Hg pressure.

The rate of glomerular filtration is determined by renal blood flow. Under normal circumstances 25 per cent of the cardiac output circulates through the kidneys. The rate of glomerular filtration is estimated to be about 130 ml per minute; 180 to 200 liters of this filtrate is formed in a 24-hour period.

In health, the glomerular filtrate tends to remain constant. If an elevation of systemic systolic pressure occurs, the afferent glomerular arteriole constricts, keeping glomerular blood flow constant. When systemic pressure falls, the afferent arteriole dilates and the efferent arteriole constricts, maintaining sufficient glomerular capillary pressure to permit filtration. Insufficient renal blood flow decreases glomerular filtration.

Reabsorption of a vast amount of the glomerular filtrate is the function of the tubule. When you consider the fact that urine passes into the bladder at the rate of 1 to 2 ml per minute, it is obvious that the reabsorption of about 98 per cent of the glomerular filtrate is accomplished by the work of the tubular cells.

ANTIDIURETIC HORMONE (ADH)

The role that the endocrine system plays in water conservation and excretion is complicated. Several hormonal agents contribute to the maintenance of a balance between water conservation and excretion. The role that many of these agents play is as yet not fully understood. Water conservation, or antidiuresis, is the function of the antidiuretic hormone. This hormone is formed by neurosecretory cells within the hypothalamus.[8] This substance then passes down via the pituitary stalk into the posterior lobe of the pituitary (pars nervosa), where it is stored and released as needed. The site of storage is within nerve endings in the pars distalis. These endings are in juxtaposition to capillaries into which the hormone can be rapidly released in response to the appropriate stimulus.[9]

Recent experiments[10] suggest that ADH may have three major functions in salt and water homeostasis: (1) antidiuretic activity, (2) adrenocorticotropic hormone (ACTH) releasing activity, and (3) direct stimulating effect on the adrenal cortex. To date, the best-defined role of the ADH is the promotion of renal tubular reabsorption of water. Suppression of ADH secretion is essential for the production of water diuresis and the elimination of excess water. Approximately 80 per cent of the water filtered through the glomerulus is reabsorbed through the proximal convoluted tubule and loop of Henle by the process of passive diffusion consequent to the reabsorption of solutes (obligatory reabsorption). In the distal convoluted tubules and beginning of the collecting tubules water is reabsorbed only when ADH is present to increase the permeability of the tubular membrane to water (facultative reabsorption). As a result of this hormonal activity, more water is reabsorbed and the volume of urine is reduced.

The mechanism of control of ADH secretion is due to slight changes in the osmotic pressure of the blood circulating around neurosecretory cells within the hypothalamus. As a result of these osmotic pressure changes, the hypothalamus is stimulated to release or to inhibit the release of the antidiuretic principle from storage in the pars nervosa. Cells that are sensitive to very slight osmotic pressure changes in the blood circulating around them are known as osmoreceptors. The anterior lobe of the pituitary (pars distalis) also affects water metabolism directly by secreting a diuretic principle (DH) as well as indirectly through ACTH secretion.[11]

There are two other endocrine factors of importance in diuresis: an adrenocortical hormone, aldosterone, and thyroid hormone. When excessive aldosterone is present, there is increased sodium reabsorption in the proximal tubule with resulting decrease in urine volume. This leads to fluid retention.

Thyroid hormone may increase diuresis by enhancing glomerular filtration and renal blood flow.

REFERENCES

1. BLAND, JOHN H.: *Clinical Metabolism of Body Water and Electrolytes.* W. B. Saunders, Philadelphia, 1963.
2. CLARKE, H. J.: *Ion Transport Across Membranes.* Academic Press, New York, 1954.
3. USSING, H. H.: "Transport Through Biological Membranes," *Ann Rev Physiol,* **15**:1, 1953.
4. DRINKER, CARL, and JEFFERY, J.: *Lymphatics, Lymph and Lymphoid Tissue.* Harvard University Press, Cambridge, 1937.
5. NEWBURGH, L. H., and JOHNSTON, M. W.: "Insensible Loss of Water." *Physiol Rev,* **22**:1, 1942.
6. CONN, J. W.: "Electrolyte Composition of Sweat: Clinical Implications as an Index of Adrenocorticotropic Function." *Arch Intern Med,* **83**:416, 1949.
7. GAMBLE, J. L.: *Chemical Anatomy, Physiology and Pathology of Extracellular Fluids.* Harvard University Press, Cambridge, 1947.
8. SCHARRER, E., and SCHARRER, B.: "Hormones Produced by Neurosecretory Cells." *Recent Progr Hormone Res,* **10**:183, 1954.
9. CHALMERS, T. M.: "The Pituitary Gland" in *Clinical Physiology,* ed. by Campbell, E. J. Moran; Dickinson, C. J.; and Slater, J. D. H., 2nd ed. F. A. Davis, Philadelphia, 1963.
10. SAWYER, WILBUR H.; MUNSICK, R.; and VAN DYK, R. B.: "Antidiuretic Hormone." *Circulation,* **21**:1037, 1960.
11. KUPPERMAN, HERBERT S. H.: *Human Endocrinology,* Vol. 1. F. A. Davis, Philadelphia, 1963.

ADDITIONAL READINGS

ADOLPH, E. A.; BARKER, JANE; and HOY, PATRICIA: "Multiple Factors in Thirst," *Amer J Physiol,* **78**:538–49, 1954.
ASHLEY, FRANKLIN, and LOVE, HORACE: *Fluid and Electrolyte Therapy.* J. B. Lippincott, Philadelphia, 1954.
BROOKS, STEWART: *Basic Facts of Body Water and Ions.* Springer, New York, 1960.
ELKINGTON, J. R., and DANOWSKI, T. S.: *The Body Fluids.* Williams and Wilkins, Baltimore, 1955.
GILMAN, A.: "The Relation Between Blood Osmotic Pressure, Fluid Distribution and Volume of Water Intake," *Amer J Physiol,* **120**:320, 1937.
GOTTSCHALK, C.: "Osmotic Concentration and Dilution in the Mammalian Nephron," *Circulation,* **21**:861, 1960.
HARDY, JAMES P.: *Fluid Therapy.* Lea and Febiger, Philadelphia, 1954.
HIGGINS, J. A.; CODE, C. F.; and ORVIS, A. L.: "The Influence of Motility on the Rate of Absorption of Sodium and Water from the Small Intestines of Healthy Persons," *Gastroenterology,* **31**:708, 1954.
HILTON, JAMES G.: "Adrenocortical Activity of ADH," *Circulation,* **21**:1038, 1960.

KEITEL, HANS: *The Pathophysiology and Treatment of Body Fluid Disturbances.* Appleton-Century-Crofts, New York, 1962.

KROGH, A.: *Anatomy and Physiology of Capillaries,* rev. ed. Yale University Press, New Haven, Conn., 1929.

LE QUESNE, L. P.: "The Body Fluids" in *Clinical Physiology,* ed. by Campbell, E. J. Moran; Dickinson, C. J.; and Slater, J. D. H., 2nd ed. F. A. Davis, Philadelphia, 1963.

STATLAND, HARRY: *Fluids and Electrolytes in Practice.* J. B. Lippincott, Philadelphia, 1954.

STEELE, J. M.: "Body Water," *Amer Med,* 9:141, 1950.

SYMPOSIA OF THE SOCIETY FOR EXPERIMENTAL BIOLOGY, VIII: *Active Transport and Secretion.* Academic Press, New York, 1954.

WELT, LOUIS, J.: "Water Balance in Health and Disease" in Duncan, G. C.: *Diseases of Metabolism,* 4th ed. W. B. Saunders, Philadelphia, 1959.

WOLF, A. V.: "Thirst," *Scient Amer,* 194:70, 1956.

———: "Body Water," *Scient Amer,* 199:125, 1958.

CHAPTER 2

The Electrolytes in Body Fluids

MAJOR differences exist in the composition of the extracellular and intracellular fluids. Those substances that are the components of extracellular fluid are, today, more completely understood than those that comprise intracellular fluids because extracellular fluid is the less complex fluid and is more readily available for analysis.

The Electrolytes in Extracellular Fluid

BLOOD SERUM

The commonly accepted normal ranges of the concentration in blood serum are:

Cations	
Sodium	135–147 mEq/liter
Potassium	3.5–5.5 mEq/liter
Calcium	4.5–5.5 mEq/liter
Magnesium	1.5–3.0 mEq/liter

Anions	
Chloride	98–106 mEq/liter
Bicarbonate	26–30 mEq/liter
Phosphate and sulfate	2–5 mEq/liter
Organic acids	3–6 mEq/liter
Proteins	15–19 mEq/liter

The approximate average sum of the concentration of all the cations is 150 mEq per liter. This is considered to be identical with the total anion concentration. As a result blood serum as a whole situation is electrically neutral.

Interstitial Fluid

The substances present in the interstitial fluid are the same as those found in plasma with one major exception. In the interstitial fluid the concentration of proteins is much lower; ordinarily the large protein molecules are unable to diffuse through the capillary endothelium. The concentration of the diffusible ions, such as sodium and chloride, differs from the concentration of these ions in plasma. This is because in the interstitial fluid a portion of these ions is chemically bound to protein.

The Electrolytes in Intracellular Fluid

The following average composition of muscle cell fluid is inferred:[1]

Cations
Potassium	150 mEq/liter
Magnesium	40 mEq/liter
Sodium	10 mEq/liter

Anions
Phosphates	140 mEq/liter
Proteinates	40 mEq/liter
Bicarbonate	10 mEq/liter
Sulfates	10 mEq/liter

Individual Electrolytes of Body Fluids

The electrolytes in the body fluids are derived from minerals. These minerals are contained in the foods we eat and are well distributed in food. The normal daily requirements of these elements are increased during the stress imposed by illness. This is especially significant during the period of anabolism that follows the catabolic phase of injury and illness, as well as in the physiological anabolic periods, such as growth.

Sodium

SODIUM INTAKE AND REQUIREMENTS

Sodium is the dominant cation of extracellular fluid. Approximately two thirds of the total exchangeable sodium is in the extracellular fluid, and the remaining third is divided between intracellular fluid and bone.[2] Sodium is ingested as it occurs in food and as sodium chloride or other sodium salts added to food in cooking, in preserving, and at the table. The use of sodium to add palatability to foods is largely determined by taste. Sodium chloride is needed for both its positive and negative ions. In the United States the customary intake of sodium is estimated to be 3 to 7 gm per person per day, or the equivalent of 7.6 to 18 gm table salt per day.[3] This intake is considered to be more than sufficient for the normal daily requirements. Requirements of sodium, as well as of potassium and chloride, have not been established, since deficiencies are rarely encountered under usual conditions. The sodium ingested is rapidly distributed in the extracellular fluid.

FUNCTIONS OF SODIUM

The primary physiological function of sodium is the control of the distribution of water throughout the body. Sodium accomplishes this function because it is the chief factor in maintaining osmotic equilibrium between extracellular and intracellular fluid compartments.

Sodium ions increase the permeability of cell membranes, a function that these ions share with potassium. Sodium, in conjunction with other extracellular ions, functions (1) as a buffer base in conjunction with bicarbonate and phosphate, (2) in the conduction of nerve impulses, (3) in the maintenance of neuromuscular irritability, and (4) in muscle contractility, especially the control of heart muscle contractility.

RENAL AND HORMONAL ASPECTS OF SODIUM METABOLISM

The kidney has evolved an elaborate mechanism for the conservation, or release, of sodium. By this mechanism the kidney is the chief organ that maintains the osmolarity of extracellular fluid within narrow limits. Through this control of the sodium content of the body the kidney is capable of preventing sudden changes in the water content of the body. The principal means by which the kidney controls the amount of sodium excreted in urine is by altering the amount of this ion reabsorbed in the renal tubules. The main factor initiating a change in sodium excretion or reabsorption is an alteration of the fluid content of the body. A decrease in circulating blood volume, intracellular volume, or total body water leads to an increase in sodium reabsorption with a concomitant increase in water reabsorption. This homeostatic mechanism thus is a prime factor in the maintenance of fluid volume. This mechanism is triggered into action by hormonal factors. The principal hormone involved is probably a mineralocorticoid of the adrenal cortex. This humoral agent is aldosterone.

Aldosterone has been found to be a potent, naturally occurring salt-retaining hormone. It acts on the renal tubules to promote sodium retention and potassium excretion.

The secretion of aldosterone is dependent on the sodium and potassium levels in the blood stream as well as the degree of hydration of body tissues. Adrenocorticotropic hormone (ACTH) is required to maintain the adrenal synthesis of aldosterone at a high level.[4]

Calcium

Calcium is essential to the proper functioning of all cells. Approximately 99 per cent of the total body calcium is concentrated in bone. A relatively minor, yet physiologically important, fraction of calcium is in other tissues and extracellular fluid. The calcium in blood is present in three forms: ionized, protein-bound, and complexed. Only the ionized form is physiologically active.

CALCIUM INTAKE AND REQUIREMENTS

The body is in constant need of calcium ions. Although modern diets vary considerably, about 800 mg of calcium is consumed daily.[5] The amount of calcium retained within the body depends not only on calcium intake, but also on the amount absorbed from the gastrointestinal tract and the amount excreted. Calcium absorption from the intestines is largely determined by the availability of vitamin D. Absorption is further affected by other factors, such as the pH of the upper duodenum (where the bulk of calcium is absorbed) and the amount of magnesium present. Calcium salts are more soluble at acid levels of pH than at alkaline levels. Calcium forms insoluble, and thus inabsorbable, salts with some of the anions in the intestinal tract. Owing to these factors much of the ingested calcium may not be absorbed. The intestinal elimination of calcium is increased by a lack of vitamin D. Because of the variability of the amount of calcium absorbed, perhaps only 300 mg of the amount ingested may be absorbed. Because of this variability in the amount absorbed and eliminated it is preferable to have an oversupply in the diet. Recommended daily allowances are:[3]

Adults	0.8 gm
Infants and growing children	0.7–1.4 gm
Second and third trimesters of pregnancy and lactation	1.3–1.5 gm

Calcium is not widely distributed in our natural foods. It is the one nutrient whose adequacy in the diet is directly related to the inclusion of a specific food, milk, in the daily meals. Milk and milk products contribute the major share of calcium available to us from the foods we eat. Dairy products contribute three fourths of the calcium in our food supply. A quart of cow's milk contains about 1.2 gm of calcium.

Vegetables and fruits provide the second best source of calcium. Fruits are somewhat lower in their calcium content. The amount that can be eaten at one time qualifies the importance of the food as a source of calcium.

FUNCTIONS OF CALCIUM

Calcium ions serve the following functions: (1) they decrease neuromuscular irritability, (2) they decrease capillary membrane permeability, (3) they are required for normal muscle contractility, (4) they are necessary for proper transmission of nerve impulses, and (5) they are essential to the clotting of blood. Calcium salts, particularly calcium phosphate, are required for the building of bones and teeth.

Bone and the Extracellular Fluid

Understanding electrolyte homeostasis requires knowledge of the relationship that bony tissue plays in the constancy of the electrolyte composition of the body. Although the various electrolytes are considered separately, in physiological reality, the functions of the electrolytes are interrelated and interdependent.

Bone plays a considerable role in maintaining the constancy of the electrolyte composition of the body. Besides containing nearly all the body's calcium and about 88 per cent of its phosphorus, bone contains the following approximate amounts of electrolytes:

Magnesium	58 per cent
Sodium	33–40 per cent
Potassium	6 per cent

By themselves these figures have little physiological relevance. What is of importance is the amount of these minerals that is freely and readily available from bone stores to contribute to the homeostasis of the electrolyte composition of body fluids. Through certain research techniques (isotope dilution studies) it has been shown that about 30 per cent of bone sodium and about 20 per cent of the magnesium is readily available.[2] About 0.2 per cent to about 1.8 per cent of the total bone calcium is available. These figures represent a considerable amount of the total exchangeable calcium in the body, an amount sufficient to offset acute decreases in blood calcium levels.

The Parathyroid Glands and Calcium Homeostasis

Parathormone (PTH), the hormone of the parathyroid glands, functions in the control of the regulation of the concentration of calcium and phosphorus in plasma and bone. In order to prevent depletion of skeletal reserves, dietary calcium must be sufficient. Furthermore, efficient intestinal absorption of this mineral must take place. PTH maintains a normal calcium equilibrium by (1) increasing intestinal absorption of calcium, (2) increasing renal tubular reabsorption of calcium, and (3) increasing resorption from the available pool in bone.[4]

The factors influencing the release of PTH are related to variations in plasma concentration of calcium and phosphorus. Specifically, increased levels of plasma calcium will inhibit secretion and release of PTH and promote urinary calcium excretion. Consequently, serum calcium levels will return to their normal value. Conversely, decreased serum calcium levels will stimulate the release of PTH; this promotes increased bone resorption of calcium and increased intestinal absorption of calcium. These actions will raise the serum calcium concentration to normal.

Potassium

POTASSIUM INTAKE AND REQUIREMENTS

Potassium is the dominant intracellular cation and the most abundant cation in the body. It is the ion that cells tolerate.

Potassium is derived from animal or vegetable cells taken in food or drink. It is readily available as it is present in high concentrations in almost all foods. Only limited data are available on the potassium requirements of man.[3] An intake of 0.8 to 1.3 gm per day has been estimated to be near the minimal potassium need. Usual diets in the United States contain from 0.8 to 1.5 gm potassium per 1000 calories.[3] Potassium ions are readily absorbed from the intestinal tract and parenteral sites of administration. The intestinal absorption of potassium is nearly complete, and normally the feces contain very little potassium. After the absorption of potassium, the ion first gains access to the extracellular fluid. From this site it rapidly enters cells, particularly those of liver and skeletal and cardiac muscle.

FUNCTIONS OF POTASSIUM

No other ion can functionally replace potassium in the cell. Therefore, the functional integrity of the cell is dependent on potassium. Potassium plays an integral part in many physiological processes. This ion is the chief regulator of intracellular osmolarity and electroneutrality, a role analogous to that of sodium in extracellular fluid. The intracellular concentration of potassium is necessary for the action of certain enzyme systems associated with the production of energy for cellular work, and it is required for cellular growth. Potassium supplies the cations for the organic anions essential for the composition of protoplasm. Growing children must be in positive potassium balance in order to form new tissue of normal electrolyte composition. Potassium is concerned with the conduction of nerve impulses, and nerve fibers are especially rich in this element. Nerve impulses may be blocked by either high or low concentrations of potassium. Skeletal muscle function is related to potassium metabolism; during muscle cell contraction potassium moves out of the muscle cell in exchange for sodium. The significance of this movement of ions is not clear, but it seems to be connected with the contractile process.[6] In high concentrations potassium has a depressant action on the myocardium, so that the heart stops in diastole. With low potassium levels the opposite effect obtains, and the heart stops in systole. Glycogen deposition cannot take place in liver cells unless potassium ions are present.

RENAL EXCRETION OF POTASSIUM

Excretion of potassium is predominantly via the kidney. There is no elaborate renal mechanism for potassium conservation and release such as has evolved for sodium. In order to maintain potassium balance the daily amount excreted in urine should roughly approximate the amount consumed in the diet. Two processes are involved in the renal excretion of potassium, viz., reabsorption in the proximal tubule and secretion of the ion into the distal tubule. Normally, the amount present in urine represents approximately 10 per cent of the amount filtered by the glomeruli. Adrenocortical steroids are believed to increase tubular excretion of potassium in exchange for sodium.[7]

Magnesium

MAGNESIUM INTAKE AND REQUIREMENTS

Magnesium is present in abundance in food. Green plants contain large amounts, since it is the essential metal in chlorophyll. It is virtually impossible to have a magnesium deficiency on an ordinary diet. The normal magnesium requirement is estimated to be about 200 to 300 mg per day.[3]

Magnesium is absorbed with difficulty from the intestinal tract. Factors influencing magnesium absorption are the same as those for calcium. An acid reaction in the duodenum enhances absorption.

Most of the ingested magnesium is excreted in the feces, but a small fraction is eliminated by the kidneys. The stool content varies with the dietary content. PTH may play a role in the urinary excretion of magnesium.[1]

FUNCTION OF MAGNESIUM

Magnesium is essential for the functional integrity of the neuro-muscular system. It exerts a sedative action on this system, an effect that is antagonized by calcium. Magnesium is required for the enzymatic action involved in intracellular energy transformations of phosphate bonds. The proper ratio of sodium, potassium, calcium, and magnesium is of importance in regulating the excitability of many, if not all, cells.

Chloride

CHLORIDE INTAKE AND REQUIREMENTS

Chloride is the chief anion of extracellular fluid. The intake of this ion occurs when the salt, sodium chloride, is added to food. Intake is closely related to the amount of sodium in foods, body fluids, and excretions. The intake is the same as for sodium.

FUNCTIONS OF CHLORIDE

The highest concentration of chloride ions occurs in the parietal cells of the stomach, where it is required for the secretion of gastric hydrochloric acid. The major function of this ion is the part it plays in the osmolarity of respiratory gases in the blood in the phenomenon of the "chloride shift." (See Glossary.)

Chloride is excreted chiefly by the kidney, mainly as the salt, sodium chloride. Reabsorption of approximately 80 per cent of the amount filtered by the glomeruli occurs in the proximal tubule as a passive process along with the reabsorption of sodium.

Phosphorus

PHOSPHORUS INTAKE AND REQUIREMENTS

The phosphate ion is the dominant anion of intracellular fluid. Deficiencies are uncommon, and diets that are adequate in content of calcium are likely to contain more than the necessary amounts of phosphorus. In ordinary diets, the phosphorus intake of adults is approximately one and one-half times that of calcium. In general, it is safe to assume that if calcium and protein needs are met through ordinary diets, the phosphorus requirement will also be met, because the foods richest in calcium and protein are also the best sources of phosphorus.

FUNCTIONS OF PHOSPHORUS

The phosphate ion serves a variety of functions in the body. About 88 per cent of all the body's phosphorus is contained in the skeleton as the salt, calcium phosphate. This concentration as a bone salt gives rigidity to bone. Phosphorus is essential to the acid-base equilibrium of body fluids. In the intermediary metabolism of carbohydrate, the first step in the production of glycogen is the reaction of glucose with adenosine triphosphate (ATP), an energy-rich compound widely distributed in animal and plant tissues. The phosphate compounds ATP and adenosine diphosphate (ADP) take part in many biochemical reactions to provide energy for cellular work.

Sulfur

Little is known at this time about the requirements for sulfur. The sulfate ion does not penetrate cell membranes. This ion appears in the cellular fluid because it is a constituent of the amino acids methionine and cystine. It is manufactured in the cells from these amino acids in the course of intracellular metabolism. Sulfur is derived from these amino acids. Sulfur-containing amino acids are believed to be involved in mitosis, building of tissue proteins, and wound healing.[8]

REFERENCES

1. BLAND, JOHN H.: *Clinical Metabolism of Body Water and Electrolytes.* W. B. Saunders, Philadelphia, 1963.
2. EDELMAN, T. S., and LEIBMAN, J.: "Anatomy of Body Water and Electrolytes," *Amer J Med,* **27**:256, 1959.
3. NATIONAL RESEARCH COUNCIL PUBLICATION 1146: Dietary Allowances, 6th ed. rev. Washington, D. C., 1963.
4. KUPPERMAN, HERBERT S.: *Endocrinology,* Vol. 1. F. A. Davis, Philadelphia, 1963.

5. CAMPBELL, E. J. MORAN; DICKINSON, C. J.; and SLATER, J. D. H.: *Clinical Physiology*, 2nd ed. F. A. Davis, Philadelphia, 1963.
6. FENN, W. O.: "The Role of Potassium in Physiologic Processes," *Physiol Rev*, **20**:377, 1940.
7. RELMAN, A. S., and SCHWARTZ, W. B.: "The Kidney in Potassium Depletion," *Amer J Med*, **24**:764, 1958.
8. SHOHOL, A. T.: "Mineral Metabolism," Am Chem Soc Monograph Series No. 82, *The Chemical Catalog*. New York, 1940.

ADDITIONAL READINGS

AUGUST, J. T.; NELSON, D. H.; and THORN, G. H.: "Response of Normal Subjects to Large Amounts of Aldosterone," *J Clin Invest*, **37**:549, 1958.
BROOKS, STEWART: *Basic Facts of Body Water and Ions*. Springer, New York, 1960.
GAMBLE, J. L.: *Clinical Anatomy, Physiology and Pathology of Extracellular Fluid*, 6th ed. Harvard University Press, Cambridge, 1958.
GUZMAN, BARRON E. S.: *Modern Trends in Physiology and Bio-chemistry*. Academic Press, New York, 1952.
HARRISON, H. E., and HARRISON, HELEN C.: "Renal Excretion of Phosphate in Relation to Vitamin D and Parathyroid Hormone," *J Clin Invest*, **20**:47, 1941.
HILLS, A. G.; CHALMERS, T. M.; WEBSTER, G. D., JR.; and ROSENTHAL, O.: "Adrenal Cortical Regulation of Distribution of Water and Electrolytes in Human Body," *J Clin Invest*, **32**:1236, 1953.
LUETSCHER, J. A., JR., and CURTIS, R. H.: "Aldosterone: Observations on the Regulation of Sodium and Potassium Balance," *Ann Intern Med*, **43**:658, 1955.
MANERY, J. F.: "Water and Electrolyte Metabolism," *Physiol Rev*, **34**:334, 1954.
MUDGE, GILBERT H.: "Potassium Imbalance," *Bull N Y Acad Med*, **29**:846, 1951.
NATIONAL RESEARCH COUNCIL PUBLICATION 325: *Sodium Restricted Diets: The Rationale, Complications and Practical Aspects of Their Use*. Washington, D. C., July, 1954.
PITTS, R. F., and ALEXANDER, R. S.: "The Renal Reabsorptive Mechanism for Inorganic Phosphate in Normal and Acidotic Dogs," *Amer J Physiol*, **142**:684, 1944.
SHERMAN, H. C.: *Calcium and Phosphorus in Foods and Nutrition*. Columbia University Press, New York, 1950.
———: *Chemistry of Foods and Nutrition*, 8th ed. Macmillan, New York, 1952.
WACKER, W. E., and VALLEE, B. L.: "Magnesium Metabolism," *New Eng J Med*, **259**:431, 1958.
WIDDOWSON, E. M.; MCCANCE, R. B.; and SPRAY, C. M.: "Chemical Composition of the Human Body," *Clin Pediat*, **10**;113, 1951.

CHAPTER 3

Acid-Base Regulation

THE healthy body maintains a remarkable and precise balance between the various electrolytes in the body fluids. The most striking evidence of this is illustrated by the relative constancy of the balance between the hydrogen ion–hydroxyl ion concentration of body fluids. It is no small achievement to maintain a concentration of these particular ions within the range of tolerance for survival and more especially within the narrow range that permits normal function. Our lives are spent fighting off the ever-present threat of a metabolic acidosis. Large and varying amounts of acids are produced as a result of cellular metabolism. In addition, varying amounts of acids and alkalis are introduced by way of the mouth. The end products of metabolism include inorganic and organic acids—carbonic, sulfuric, phosphoric, lactic, and others. These acids are rapidly neutralized by bases present in the blood and tissue fluids, chiefly sodium bicarbonate. As a result of these neutralization reactions, inorganic and organic salts and carbon dioxide are formed. Most of these salts are eliminated by the kidneys, and the carbon dioxide is eliminated by the lungs.

Inasmuch as all mammals are acid-producers, the healthy functioning of all cells is closely related to the hydrogen ion concentration [H^+] in extracellular and cellular fluids. At the present time far less is known about the concentration of hydrogen ions within the cells than is known about the concentration of this ion in extracellular fluids. Therefore, this discussion will be limited almost exclusively to the acid-base regulation in extracellular fluids.

Definitions

The reaction of a solution is acid when the concentration of hydrogen ions exceeds the concentration of hydroxyl ions; it is

30

alkaline when the concentration of hydroxyl ions exceeds that of hydrogen ions; and neutral when the concentrations of both are equal.

The terminology used herein is according to Bronsted and is based on the hydrogen ion:[1]

1. The positively charged hydrogen ion is a proton, the atomic nucleus that remains after a hydrogen atom has given its one electron.
2. An acid is a hydrogen donor—something that gives hydrogen ions to a solution and makes it more acid.
3. A base is a hydrogen acceptor—something that takes or accepts hydrogen ions from the solution, rendering it less acid.

The more readily an acid relinquishes its protons, the stronger it is as an acid, and the more readily a base accepts protons, the stronger it is as a base. Free protons do not exist as such in solution; they react with molecules of water to form hydronium ions, H_3O^+. As these molecules are reactive by virtue of their extra proton, they are expressed in terms of pH.

At any temperature the product of the concentration of hydrogen ions and the product of the concentration of hydroxyl ions in a solution in water are constant. Because of this fixed and definite quality the reaction of a solution can be defined precisely by specifying the $[H^+]$ *only*. With the exception of very acid solutions, the $[H^+]$ is so small that it can only be expressed in mols per liter in inconveniently small numbers.

For example, pure water at 25°C contains 0.0000001 mol of hydrogen ions per liter. Water at this temperature also contains 0.0000001 mol of hydroxyl ions per liter. The $[H^+]$ multiplied by the $[OH^-]$ is always equal to the exceedingly small value of 0.00000000000001. Thus:

$$[H^+] \times [OH^-] = 10^{-14}$$

Such small concentrations are expressed in the pH notation, by changing the negative exponent (in this example 10^{-14}) to the positive power of 10. pH is defined as the negative common logarithm (base of 10) of the hydrogen ion concentration, or

$$pH = -\log [H^+]$$

Frequently pH is defined as the positive power on the basis of ten (or the positive logarithm) of the reciprocal of the $[H^+]$ of the solution. The pH value is the same under either definition. In the latter definition the computation is made in terms of the reciprocal of the [H$^+$] of the solution, then converted to the actual [H$^+$] value. For example;

$$\frac{1}{[H^+]} = \frac{1}{10^5} = 10^5 \ldots \text{pH} = 5$$

The use of the pH values follows the rules of logarithmic calculation: every change of the pH by one unit corresponds to a change in [H$^+$] by the factor of 10.

The pH of pure water is 7.0; this is also the pH of neutrality. If an acid is added to the solution, the [H$^+$] will increase and there will be a greater number of hydrogen ions with a smaller exponent number. The pH of acid solutions is less than seven and that of basic solutions is greater than seven.

Table 1

THE RELATIONSHIP BETWEEN pH AND
HYDROGEN ION AND mEq/L

pH	H$^+$	mEq/L
1.0	1×10^{-1}	100
2.0	1×10^{-2}	10
3.0	1×10^{-3}	1
4.0	1×10^{-4}	0.1
5.0	1×10^{-5}	0.01
6.0	1×10^{-6}	0.001
7.0	1×10^{-7}	0.0001
8.0	1×10^{-8}	0.00001

Substances that neither donate nor accept hydrogen ions are neither acids nor bases. Acids and bases are *not* the same as anions and cations. For example, an acid may be electrically neutral, an anion, or a cation:

$$HCl \rightleftarrows H^+ = Cl^-$$
Electrically neutral

$$H_2PO_4^- \rightleftarrows HPO_4^= + H^+$$
Anion

$$NH_4 \rightleftarrows H^+ + NH_3$$
Cation

Substances such as the sodium ion, which are often referred to clinically as bases, are in chemical usage neither acids nor bases, because they can neither donate nor accept hydrogen ions.

The Normal Reaction of Body Fluids

The plasma of arterial blood in healthy persons ranges from pH 7.36 to pH 7.44. pH 7.40 is generally accepted as the normal average value. The range compatible with survival (E.C.F.) extends from pH 6.8 to pH 7.8. The pH of infants is about 0.1 unit below the adult level.

A difference of one unit in pH implies a tenfold change in concentration. The range from pH 7.0 to pH 7.8 includes a range from 40 per cent to 250 per cent of the value normally maintained. This is greater than the range of potassium that can be tolerated and far greater than the range of tolerance for sodium. Thus tissue cells possess a greater tolerance to variations in $[H^+]$ than to variations in the concentration of any other ion.

Far less is known about the $[H^+]$ in the cellular fluid than in extracellular fluids. There is reason to believe that the fluids within the cell are more acid, with a pH around 6.9 or lower.[2] Techniques that will provide more detailed and precise study of intracellular fluid are yet to be discovered.

How Acid-Base Balance Is Regulated

The regulation of the reaction of extracellular fluid is necessary for normal cellular function. The principal acid-base regulatory mechanisms are three in number: the body buffers; respiratory regulation of oxygen–carbon dioxide exchange between cells, lungs, and external environment; and the selective elimination of ions by the kidneys. Buffering action takes place with extreme rapidity, and the respiratory response to a change in pH is also rapid, but the renal response to disposal of an excess of "fixed" cation or anion* is more gradual and may take some days to reach a maximum.

* "Fixed" anions are those such as Cl^-, SO_4-, and PO_4- which are not destroyed in metabolism and which must be excreted by the kidney. "Unfixed" anions, such as $HHCO_3-$, are disposed of as carbon dioxide and water and do not require kidney activity.

Blood and Body Buffers

When an acid is added to a solution, the $[H^+]$ increases according to the amount and strength of the acid added. If a base is added to a solution, the $[OH]$ is increased according to the amount and strength of the added base. There are solutions that will undergo very little change in the pH of the solution when considerable, although limited, amounts or strengths of acids or bases are added. Such solutions are called buffered solutions, and the components of the solution responsible for the effect are called buffers. By definition, the buffering action of a solution is the ability of that solution to take up or discharge hydrogen ions or hydroxyl ions with little change in the pH of the solution. A buffer system consists of a weakly ionized acid (or base) in equilibrium with its fully ionized salt. Such a combination resists major changes in $[H^+]$ upon the addition of a strong acid or base. For example, carbonic acid and sodium bicarbonate constitute a buffer system. If hydrochloric acid (nearly 100 per cent ionized) is added to a solution of sodium bicarbonate, the following reaction takes place:

$$H^+ + Cl^- + Na^+ + HCO_3^- \rightarrow H.HCO_{3+} + Na^+ + Cl^-$$
$$H_2CO_3 \rightleftarrows H^+ + HCO_3^-$$

Since H_2CO_3 is weakly ionized, the ultimate result is that most of the hydrogen ions exist as un-ionized H_2CO_3, and there is little change in $[H^+]$ even though many hydrogen ions have been added. In other words, the ionized sodium salt of the weak acid, carbonic, buffers the impact of the highly ionized hydrochloric acid by forming weakly ionized carbonic acid. The capacity of a buffer is limited by the number of anions available to trap hydrogen ions.

The two principal buffers in the extracellular fluid compartment are hemoglobin and the bicarbonate–carbonic acid system. The bicarbonate system is quantitatively the more important. The total buffering action of body buffers is so effective that all but five of every million hydrogen ions added are buffered.[3] Buffering action by the bicarbonate system extends also to the interstitial fluid, a volume about three times that of the plasma volume. In the cells there are a great variety of other buffers, mainly the proteinates and the monohydrogen-dihydrogen phosphate system. On the basis of volume, the cells and tissue water have about ten times the buffering action of blood alone.[4]

The buffer pairs of blood comprise:

Plasma		*Red Cells*	
Sodium bicarbonate	$NaHCO_3$	Potassium bicarbonate	$KHCO_3$
Hydrogen carbonate	H_2CO_3	Hydrogen carbonate	H_2CO_3
Sodium monohydrogen phosphate	Na_2HPO_4	Potassium monohydrogen phosphate	K_2HPO_4
Sodium dihydrogen phosphate	NaH_2PO_4	Potassium dihydrogen phosphate	KH_2PO_4
Sodium proteinate		Potassium proteinate	
Hydrogen proteinate		Hydrogen proteinate	

The sodium salts are chiefly concentrated in plasma and the potassium salts are chiefly concentrated in cells. In the blood the buffer pairs are in equilibrium with each other.

The normal concentration of H_2CO_3 is 1.37 mEq per liter. The concentration of $B.HCO_3$* is normally 27 mEq per liter.

Hence:

$$\frac{B.HCO_3}{H.HCO_3} = \frac{27}{1.37} = \frac{20}{1}$$

As long as the $\frac{B.HCO_3}{H.HCO_3}$ ratio remains 20/1, the pH of blood remains within its normal range of 7.35 to 7.44. The ratio may be 40/2 or 10/0.5 without a change in pH.

Transport of Carbon Dioxide

Carbon dioxide is produced constantly, as a result of metabolic processes, in larger amounts than any other substance. It must be transported from its site of formation at the tissue level to the lungs for elimination. Transport of carbon dioxide occurs in three forms (see below): in simple physical solution, as bicarbonate, and combined with blood proteins (chiefly hemoglobin) as carbamino compounds.

	Arterial	*Venous*
Pressure (pCO_2) in mm Hg	40 mm	46 mm
Content of CO_2 (ml/100 ml blood)	48.5 ml	52.5 ml
In solution	2.5 ml	2.8 ml
As bicarbonate	43 ml	46 ml
Carbamino compounds	3.0 ml	3.7 ml

* The letter B symbolizes the total cation Na^+, K^+, Mg^+, Ca^{++}, etc.

Approximately 2 to 3 ml of carbon dioxide is transported in simple physical solution. If all the carbon dioxide was carried in solution, the pH of blood would be 4.0, which is grossly incompatible with life. Since the pH of blood normally shows very little variation (pH 7.36 to 7.44), it is evident that the bulk of carbon dioxide must be carried in combination. Most of it is in the form of bicarbonate, in the red cells and in plasma and tissue fluids. From the cells dissolved carbon dioxide diffuses through the tissue fluid into plasma with the resulting reaction:

$$CO_2 + H_2O \leftrightarrows H_2CO_3$$

In the plasma this reaction takes place slowly. However, this same reaction proceeds very rapidly in the erythrocyte owing to the presence of an enzyme, carbonic anhydrase. In blood this enzyme is confined to the red cells. This reaction in the red cells is so rapid that it is complete by the time the blood has traversed the capillaries. Most of the carbon dioxide diffuses into the red cells, reacting with water to form carbonic acid. The carbonic acid dissociates:

$$H_2CO_3 \rightleftarrows H_2 + CO_3$$

Most of the hydrogen ions are buffered by hemoglobin. The bulk of the HCO_3^- ions diffuse from the red cell into plasma, and chloride ions enter the red cell to replace the HCO_3^- ions and thus restore ionic equilibrium. This movement of chloride ions is known as the "chloride shift." The reduced hemoglobin (HHb)* of venous blood is more capable of forming carbamino compounds than is the oxyhemoglobin (HHbO$_2$) of arterial blood. This greater affinity of reduced hemoglobin for carbon dioxide in the form of carbamino compounds enables venous blood to carry more carbon dioxide as hemoglobin. In the lungs all these processes are reversed.

To summarize events in carbon dioxide transport:

1. Carbon dioxide is continually produced within cells; therefore, its partial pressure (pCO$_2$) is highest as it diffuses into venous blood from the cells;
2. Carbon dioxide diffuses from:

$$\text{Tissue cell} \rightarrow \text{Tissue fluid} \rightarrow \text{Plasma}$$

* HHb is used to denote un-ionized hemoglobin and also to indicate that hemoglobin acts as an acid.

3. In plasma, some of the carbon dioxide enters into the following reaction:

$$CO_2 + H_2O \underset{}{\overset{slow}{\rightleftharpoons}} H_2CO_3^-$$

4. The carbonic acid ionizes and liberates hydrogen ions:

$$H_2CO_3 \rightarrow H^+ + HCO_3^-$$

In plasma these hydrogen ions are buffered by sodium bicarbonate and the plasma proteins.

5. The major portion of the carbon dioxide diffuses into the red cells where two reactions take place:

A. $$CO_2 + H_2O \xrightarrow[\text{carbonic anhydrase}]{\text{rapid}} H_2CO_3$$

B. Carbonic acid dissociates and the resulting hydrogen ions are taken up by oxyhemoglobin to form reduced hemoglobin. Reduced hemoglobin reacts with carbon dioxide to form carbamino hemoglobin:

$$HHb + CO_2 \rightarrow HHbCO_2$$

6. The HCO_3^- ions released by the prior reaction diffuse into the plasma and Cl^- ions shift into the red cells in exchange for the HCO_3^- to restore ionic equilibrium. This exchange of ions allows for the transport of many more HCO_3^- ions.

7. In the pulmonary capillaries all these reactions are reversed: carbon dioxide diffuses from blood into the alveoli, and oxygen diffuses from the alveoli into blood.

Respiratory Influences in Acid-Base Regulation

The primary pulmonary mechanism of acid-base regulation depends on the capacity of the lungs to constantly remove carbon dioxide from blood and eliminate it in the expired air. The lungs possess a greater total surface area than any other organ. Thus, the surface available for diffusion of respiratory gases is enormous. The lungs exert a strong influence on acid-base regulation. No other organ can effect such rapid changes in hydrogen ion concentration.

When venous blood reaches the pulmonary capillaries, the partial pressure of carbon dioxide is 46 mm Hg. The carbon dioxide present in the alveoli has a partial pressure of 40 mm Hg. This slight, but effective, difference in pressure facilitates the diffusion of carbon dioxide from the blood into the alveolar air, and then into the expired air. Because the expired air is moist, the carbon dioxide is in the form of H_2CO_3; as a result hydrogen ions are also eliminated.

Chemical Control of Respiration

Pulmonary ventilation is fundamentally regulated to satisfy the varying metabolic activities of the body. Respiratory neurons located in the medulla are actively concerned with pulmonary ventilation. These neurons are extremely sensitive to changes in the partial pressure of carbon dioxide in the arterial blood. An increase in arterial pCO_2 acts through the medullary centers to increase the rate of pulmonary ventilation. The increased rate will continue until sufficient carbon dioxide has been removed to return the arterial pCO_2 to 40 mm Hg. A decreased pCO_2 will either decrease or temporarily halt pulmonary ventilation. This decrease or halt will continue until there is sufficient circulating carbon dioxide to raise the pCO_2 to normal. This exquisite sensitivity of the respiratory neuron to the pCO_2 of arterial blood ensures that the excretion of carbon dioxide keeps pace with its production, and at the same time arterial pCO_2 is kept very close to 40 mm Hg. By this method the body controls the amount of volatile acid excreted.

Renal Influences on Acid-Base Regulation

Strong acids that are ingested or formed by metabolic reactions dissociate into hydrogen ions and anions. It is the hydrogen ions that lower pH; so in order to maintain a normal pH range in body fluids, the hydrogen ions and anions must be excreted. Usually the excretion of anions presents little difficulty. They exist free in the plasma and are therefore subject to glomerular filtration and to selective reabsorption and excretion by the renal tubules.

The problem of excreting hydrogen ions, however, is a real one, because these ions no longer exist as such. They have nearly all disappeared as a result of conversion to their respective salts through reactions with the body buffers. As a result hydrogen ions exist largely in the buffered state. As a result of this the kidneys do not have access to these ions, as in the case of the anions; so they must be excreted indirectly.

There are three processes available to the kidney for the excretion of acid: (1) The exchange of hydrogen ions formed in the tubule cells for sodium ions in the tubular urine is one process. In this process, the hydrogen ions derived from $H.HCO_3^-$ in the tubular cells are exchanged with sodium ions in the tubular urine. The sodium ions combine with the bicarbonate ions and are returned to the extra-cellular fluid as sodium bicarbonate. (2) The second process involves the acidification of urinary buffer salts. Since most of the bicarbonate has been removed, the principal buffer salt remaining is phosphate. In this process hydrogen ions are added to the phosphate buffer system, for example, in the conversion of Na_2HPO_4 to NaH_2PO_4. These phosphate salts are then excreted in the urine. (3) Ammonia (NH_3) is formed in the tubule cells as the result of deamination of certain amino acids. This ammonia diffuses readily into the tubular urine, where it reacts with hydrogen ions to form NH_4, which is then excreted. Approximately half the daily hydrogen ion secretion is by this method. The lungs and kidneys are referred to as the steady-state regulators. The lungs hold the responsibility for eliminating the volatile acids, and the kidneys are responsible for the excretion of the nonvolatile acids. Any factors interfering with their normal functioning will upset the balance between acid and base.

REFERENCES

1. KAUFMAN, H. E., and ROSEN, S. W.: "Clinical Acid-Base Regulation—The Bronsted Schema," *Surg Gynec Obstet*, **103**:101, 1956.
2. ROBIN, E. D., and BROMBERG, P. A.: "Editorial: Claude Bernard's Milieu Interieur Extended: Intracellular Acid-Base Relationships," *Amer J Med*, **27**:689, 1959.
3. CAMPBELL, E. J. M.: "Hydrogen Ion Regulation" in *Clinical Physiology*, by Campbell, E. J. M.; Dickinson, C. J.; and Slater, J. D. H., 2nd ed. F. A. Davis, Philadelphia, 1963.
4. ELKINGTON, J. R.: "Whole Body Buffers in the Regulation of Acid-Base Equilibrium," *Yale J Biol Med*, **29**:191, 1956.

ADDITIONAL READINGS

ASTRUP, P.; JORGENSEN, K.; ANDERSEN, O. S.; and ENGEL, K.: "Fundamentals of Acid-Base Regulation," *Lancet*, **1**:1035, 1960.

BARKER, E. S., and ELKINGTON, J. R.: "Editorial: Hydrogen Ions and Buffer Base," *Amer J Med*, **25**:1, 1958.

CHRISTENSEN, H. N.: "Anions Versus Cations," *Amer J Med*, **23**:153, 1957.

GRACE, WILLIAM J.: *Practical Clinical Management of Electrolyte Disorders*. Appleton-Century-Crofts, New York, 1960.

RELMAN, A. S.: "What Are Acids and Bases?" *Amer J Med*, **17**:435, 1954.

ROBIN, E. D., and BROMBERG, P. A.: "Of Men and Mitochrondria—Intracellular and Subcellular Acid-Base Relations," *New Eng J Med*, **265**:780, 1961.

ROBINSON, JAMES R.: *Fundamentals of Acid-Base Regulation*. Blackwell, Oxford, 1962.

SECTION II
The State of Disequilibrium

CHAPTER 4

Hydrogen Ion Imbalance

LIKE chemical sponges, the buffer systems of the body work cease-lessly to hoard or discard hydrogen ions; however, when one of the regulators fails to function adequately, the delicate range of pH is disrupted, and there follows a decrease in the bicarbonate ion or an overabundance of hydrogen ion (acidosis) or an increase in the bicarbonate ion and an underabundance of hydrogen ion (alkalosis).

Acidosis and alkalosis are further described by the nature of the hydrogen ion production. In metabolic acidosis or alkalosis the hydrogen ion is nongaseous or nonvolatile and is the product of metabolic processes. In respiratory acidosis or alkalosis the hydrogen ion is volatile or gaseous and is the product of respiratory processes. The imbalances rarely occur by themselves and are always sympto-matic of an underlying disease process. They often pose difficult problems for the diagnostician because compensatory mechanisms mask the original imbalance. For example, the patient who is hyper-ventilating and has low serum bicarbonate might have respiratory alkalosis and primary hyperventilation, or metabolic acidosis and secondary hyperventilation.[1] Clinical symptoms are evident only when compensatory mechanisms fail to establish a normal hydrogen ion range; usually, alteration in pH is so well compensated that the actual change in hydrogen ion concentration is too small to be detected. Many people have mild hydrogen ion imbalance with no visible symptoms and without any incapacitation. The magnitude of a patient's illness is proportional to the magnitude of hydrogen ion disturbance and the duration of time that the abnormal state is sustained.[2]

At this point it may be useful to summarize the defensive mech-anisms that operate to resist any change in pH.

First Line of Defense: Dilution and Buffering. Acids and bases are diluted rapidly in the extracellular fluids. Most of the hydrogen ions disappear by combining with buffer bases. The pH of plasma falls when acids are introduced into blood, but far less than if dilution did not occur and buffer bases were not readily available.

Second Line of Defense: Respiratory Compensation. Falling pH acts to stimulate the medullary respiratory centers and thus to increase pulmonary ventilation. As a result carbon dioxide is removed from the lungs at an accelerated rate and the pCO_2 falls below 40 mm Hg. This respiratory compensation reduces the concentration of carbonic acid in the plasma, thus compensating for the fall in pH. A rising pH depresses the respiratory center, and hypoventilation results. With a concomitant decrease in carbon dioxide elimination, the hypoventilatory rate will continue until the pCO_2 is reduced. This mechanism is not as precise as is the respiratory compensation for a falling pH.

Third Line of Defense: Renal Compensation. The kidneys generate new hydrogen ions equivalent to those which have been buffered in the blood and excrete them together with anions that are to be eliminated. Concurrently, the kidneys add an equivalent amount of bicarbonate to the plasma, thus maintaining the bicarbonate buffer system.

The terms used to indicate disturbances of reaction may be defined as follows:

Acidosis: A condition in which the total concentration of buffer base is reduced below normal, but the physiochemical reaction of the blood remains normal.

Alkalosis: A condition in which the total concentration of buffer base is greater than normal, but the physiochemical reaction of blood remains normal.

The terms "acidosis" and "acidemia," and "alkalosis" and "alkalemia," are frequently used interchangeably; "acidosis" and "acidemia" are used synonomously and "alkalosis" and "alkalemia" are used synonomously.

A clinically detectable acidosis or alkalosis occurs when one or more of the compensatory mechanisms fails to resist change in pH, resulting in uncompensated alkalosis or acidosis with alkalemia or acidemia. Such situations represent a threat to life. The main problem, therefore, is failure of one or more of these defensive mechanisms to the end that acidemia or alkalemia exists.

Disturbances in hydrogen ion concentration are dynamic. They consist of continuing action and reaction. Because the primary deficit is at any given time accompanied by a variety of secondary changes, clinical signs are often deceptive and the detection of an alkalosis or acidosis may not be immediately possible. By the time the blood picture alters and a true diagnosis can be made, the patient is frequently moribund and drastic measures are required to preserve life.

Essential Laboratory Studies

Determination of pH is based on a mathematical equation formulated by Henderson and Hasselbach. It shows that pH is dependent on the ratio of base to acid. Most determinations of pH in hospital laboratories are done with the aid of electrometric devices (pH meters) or by the less expensive colorimetric devices in which a dye is added to the solution in question and the color change is compared with permanent color standards.

Table 2

LABORATORY STUDIES

Tests on Blood	Normal Range	Indications
Hematocrit	41–48% packed cells	Detects hemoconcentration as volume decreases
Hemoglobin	14–16 gm/100 ml blood	or hemodilution as volume increases
Blood urea nitrogen	9–17 mg/100 ml blood	Indicates kidney function and failure to excrete end products of metabolism
Serum protein	6–8 gm/100 ml serum	Rapidly administered parenteral fluids decrease serum protein by dilution
Serum albumin	3.2–5.6 gm/100 ml serum	
Serum globulin	1.3–3.2 gm/100 ml serum	
Albumin-globulin ratio	1.5:1 to 2.5:1	Decrease in A/G ratio indicates such conditions as nephritis, malnutrition

(Continued)

Table 2   (Continued)
LABORATORY STUDIES

Blood Serum Chemistry	Normal Range, mEq/L
Sodium	135–147
Potassium	3.5–5.5
Calcium	4.5–5.5
Magnesium	1.5–3.0
Chloride	100–110
CO_2 combining power	25–30 or 56–65 vol %
CO_2 content	20–30
Nonprotein nitrogen	25–40 mg/100 ml
Proteins (total)	6.3–8.0 gm/100 ml

CARBON DIOXIDE COMBINING POWER, 25 TO 30 mEq/L OR 56 TO 65 VOL%

The carbon dioxide combining power actually indicates bicarbonate value. Normal serum combines with 56 to 65 volumes per 100 ml of carbon dioxide; that is, 100 ml of serum will absorb 56 to 65 ml of gas. An increase in carbon dioxide combining power usually indicates an alkalosis, whereas a decrease in the carbon dioxide combining power usually indicates an acidosis. The specimen of venous blood (8 ml) is drawn anaerobically either in a test tube containing mineral oil or in a vacutainer without mineral oil.

CARBON DIOXIDE CONTENT, 20 TO 30 mEq/L

Carbon dioxide content actually includes measurement of the bicarbonate ion too. It is the sum of minimal amounts of carbon dioxide and bicarbonate, plus carbonic acid. A decrease in the normal range indicates a decrease in bicarbonate, or acidosis. An elevation in normal range indicates an increase in bicarbonate, or alkalosis.

CARBON DIOXIDE PRESSURE, 35 TO 50 mm Hg

This test measures the partial pressure of carbon dioxide dissolved physically in blood and varies directly with the partial pressure of carbon dioxide in alveolar air. The partial pressure of carbon dioxide affects the direction of the equation in which $H_2CO_3 \rightarrow H_2O + CO_2$ gas. An elevated pCO_2 indicates an increased amount of carbonic acid (acidosis), whereas a low pCO_2 indicates a decreased amount of carbonic acid (alkalosis). This test is valuable in detecting respiratory imbalances.

Table 3

URINALYSIS

Tests of Urine	Normal Range	Indications
pH of freshly voided specimen	4.7–8.0	Indicates amount of hydrogen ion excreted
Specific gravity	1.003–1.030	In a dehydrated condition most water is reabsorbed by kidney. There is an increase in specific gravity
Volume of 24-hour collected specimen	1000–1500 ml	Indicates dehydration or overhydration

Average Analysis of 24-Hour Urine Specimen

Water	1200 ml
Total solids	60 gm
Ammonia	0.7 gm
Calcium	0.2 gm
Chlorides	12.0 gm
Creatine	0.03 gm
Creatinine	1.4 gm
Magnesium	0.1 gm
Potassium	2.0 gm
Sodium	4.0 gm
Urea	30.0 gm
Other solids	9.6 gm

Metabolic Acidosis

Metabolic acidosis is a condition in which there is a decrease in available base, or, in other words, a change in the extracellular bicarbonate ion concentration. The condition of excess hydrogen ion concentration, by requiring base for buffering, is also an example of metabolic acidosis. There is an increase in acid with a decrease in base.

Metabolic acidosis occurs in any clinical situation in which the patient has a decreased store of carbohydrate and in which protein and fat must be burned almost exclusively for energy. For example, in diabetic acidosis fats are excessively burned, leaving circulating ketone bodies. Every ketone molecule circulates a hydrogen ion with it, increasing the acidity of blood. These ketones require base for their excretion. The same situation occurs in such varied conditions as starvation, thyrotoxicosis, vomiting, and infections with fever. The ingestion and retention of abnormal organic acids such as salicylic acid and boric acid, paraldehyde, and methanol lead to metabolic acidosis. It has also been stipulated[3] that anesthesia in a marginally depleted individual may produce metabolic acidosis. Anesthesia causes an increase in the output of epinephrine, an increase in metabolic rate, and mobilization of hepatic glycogen as glucose and of muscle glycogen as lactic acid. This depletes carbohydrate stores and necessitates burning of fats and protein, another example of excess ketones latching on to base for excretion and causing metabolic acidosis.

In an attempt to re-establish balance, renal and respiratory mechanisms go to work. We see a person with the famous Kussmaul respiration, or breathing that is increased in rate and in depth. This breathing has also been called "acidotic" breathing and has as its purpose the blowing off of carbon dioxide. The kidneys, too, play a vital compensatory role. There is an increased hydrogen ion secretion in the tubule cells in exchange for sodium and consequent return of bicarbonate ion as sodium bicarbonate to the extracellular water and excretion of one hydrogen ion for every sodium ion recovered. This often causes a secondary metabolic alkalosis. There is also an increased ammonia secretion to exchange with salts of strong acids to recover sodium as sodium bicarbonate and excrete one hydrogen ion as ammonium chloride.[3] It is when these compensatory devices fail to keep up with the imbalance that we see true metabolic acidosis.

Clinical Signs of Metabolic Acidosis: The Patient with Diabetic Acidosis

Mr. G. is a 60-year-old man who has had diabetes mellitus for the past eight years. His illness has been controlled with tolbutamide (Orinase), 1.0 gm O.D., and with regulated diet. He has recently been hospitalized with a cerebral vascular accident. When the physician was called, Mr. G. was extremely nauseated and had been vomiting at intervals throughout the day. He complained of severe thirst and abdominal pains. His urine was tested at home and found to be 3 plus for glucose and acetone. When the physician arrived, he found a moribund patient who had dry, hot skin, parched lips, and slightly sunken eyeballs, and who was extremely weak. He was hyperventilating.

The hospital was called and instructed to be ready with available intravenous equipment, a cut-down set, a catheterization tray, and a gastric tube for stomach lavage. The rescue squad provided proper transportation for the patient.

When he arrived at the hospital, he was admitted to an intensive care unit, and a specimen of urine was obtained by the admitting nurse before the patient's clothing was removed. The nurse took the rectal temperature. Blood was drawn for immediate laboratory analysis and was found to contain:

		Normal
Glucose	300 mg %	80–100 mg %
Ketones	30 mEq/L	1 mEq/L
CO_2 content	15 mEq/L	20–30 mEq/L
Leukocytes	15,500/cu mm	4000–11,000/cu mm
Hemoglobin	17 gm %	14–16 gm/100 ml
Serum pH	7.1	7.36–7.44

Urine was examined for

sugar 3 plus	none
acetone 3 plus	none

Next 1000 ml of 0.9 per cent saline with 50 units of regular insulin was administered by vein immediately; 50 units of regular insulin was also given subcutaneously. A physical examination and history were done, followed by a bedside electrocardiogram to determine coronary status and potassium change. The nurse then assisted with gastric aspiration with warm physiological saline. This decreases the chance of aspiration of vomitus and facilitates oral intake earlier. Mr. G. had not had a bowel movement in the previous 24 hours; so a low physiological saline enema was ordered. Hourly blood pressure readings were taken to check possible impending shock. The first few hours of treatment are of vital importance to any patient in metabolic acidosis. Unless treatment is instituted promptly, the water and electrolyte losses with concomitant drop in blood volume and anuria may lead to irreversible coma. The patient must be treated in a hospital where frequent laboratory comparisons can be made.

Here is the chemical sequence that led up to this metabolic acidosis and dehydration.

1. There was a disturbance of homeostasis caused by the cerebral vascular accident. Metabolism was increased and diabetes became uncontrolled.
2. An increase in glucose in blood caused increased glucose concentration in the glomerular filtrate; the kidneys were unable to reabsorb added glucose, which caused increase loss of solution owing to excess solute load. This osmotic diuresis caused the patient to void frequently (polyuria) and complain of extreme thirst.
3. An increased tonicity of the extracellular fluid drew fluid out of cells with potassium and magnesium (cations) and phosphate (anion). Though the hematocrit level may appear normal, there is actually cellular dehydration.
4. With the excessive burning of fats and protein for energy, there was a drastic increase in circulating ketones that must combine with fixed base for their excretion. There was a further loss of sodium with continued cellular and extracellular dehydration.
5. Marked dehydration decreased blood volume, which in turn decreased the amount of blood through the kidney, causing further retention of organic acid wastes, sulfates, and phosphates. The amount of potassium circulating in the blood increased to dangerous levels. This decreased blood volume may lead to shock and irreversible water and electrolyte losses. [1]

Let us take another look at the symptoms stemming from this sequence of events. We see a patient who looks very sick, is nauseated, and is so weak he can barely sit up. What began as polyuria has now become oliguria, with scanty, highly concentrated urine. His tongue is furry and his eyes appear sunken, with eyeballs soft from decrease in fluid. His mucous membranes are dry. He is hyperventilating.

THE RATIONALE OF TREATMENT

The immediate goals for the patient in metabolic acidosis are to re-establish adequate blood volume, to provide sufficient insulin to re-establish carbohydrate oxidation, and to correct the extracellular and intracellular losses of water and electrolytes. This is done primarily by early, liberal administration of insulin and some fluid. Rather than attempting to replace total quantities of lost fluid, the object is to allow the body's own homeostatic mechanism to take over and thereby prevent the possibility of overloading the circulatory system.

Bland[3] has described the three major stages of treatment (Table 4).

Table 4
WATER AND ELECTROLYTE THERAPY IN DIABETIC COMA: SIMPLIFIED, ADEQUATE REGIMEN*

Hours of Treatment	Solution	Added Electrolytes
0 to 2	1000 to 2000 ml of 0.9% NaCl or 1000 ml 0.9% NaCl plus 960 ml 0.6% NaCl	None other than potassium rarely 40 ml (40 mEq) 1.0 molar Na lactate or $NaHCO_3$ added to second IV
2 to 6	1000 to 2000 ml 0.6% NaCl containing $\rightarrow$ Change to 5% D/W 200 ml/hour if blood sugar approaching normal	40–80 ml 1.0 molar Na lactate or $NaHCO_3$ plus 2 ampuls (40 mEq) KCL or 2 ampuls (50 mEq) K phosphate (K_2HPO_4 2 gm, KH_2PO_4 0.4 gm)
6 to 24	100–120 ml orally when tolerated of broth, dilute orange juice, etc. If not tolerated, withhold; give 1000 ml 0.9% NaCl or D/W at 10–15 gm/hour if blood sugar low or normal	KCL (40 mEq) or K phosphate (50 mEq)

*FROM Bland, John H., *Clinical Metabolism of Body Water and Electrolytes*. W. B. Saunders, Philadelphia, 1963. Reprinted by permission of the publisher.

It is important to know the blood glucose level, the size of the patient, and the length of time he has had diabetes. Usually more insulin is needed for the patient with long-standing disease. Some persons are found to be insulin resistant if they have had diabetes for a long time and require larger amounts. A very few persons are found to be allergic to large quantities of insulin; this is the only reason part of the insulin is given by vein, part subcutaneously. When the severe hyperglycemia and glycosuria are brought under control, there may be a temporary insulin edema that disappears if kidney function is adequate.[1] The patient states that he feels bloated and has blurred vision, and a gain in weight is noted. Tetany due to hypocalcemia may complicate the treatment of metabolic acidosis. The patient with severe acidosis who is treated with sodium bicarbonate may develop hypocalcemic tetany since an increase in hydrogen ion concentration results in increased binding of calcium by protein with resulting hypocalcemia. This occurs more often in patients treated with high sodium and low potassium intake than in patients treated with moderate amounts of each ion.[4] Calcium gluconate may be administered to help prevent hypocalcemia.[5]

Respiratory Acidosis

Respiratory acidosis is a condition in which there is an increase in extracellular carbonic acid concentration or a gain in volatile, gaseous carbon dioxide. Origin of the condition is pulmonary. Such acidosis may occur in any condition in which the ventilatory efficiency of the lungs is diminished. Some common causative conditions include emphysema, bronchiectasis, pneumothorax, hemothorax, inadequate ventilation during surgery, bronchial asthma, bronchial pneumonia, neuromuscular diseases such as poliomyelitis, pulmonary fibrosis, lung edema, depression of respiratory neurons caused by drug intoxication, acute alcoholism, overbreathing of carbon dioxide, and wounds or burns of the upper respiratory tract. Respiratory acidosis is not seen as frequently as metabolic acidosis.

Compensatory mechanisms attempt to re-establish carbonic acid-base bicarbonate ratio of 1:20 through blood buffers, pulmonary mechanisms, and renal mechanisms. Through the movement of chloride ions from the plasma into red cells (chloride shift), bicarbonate ions are released to neutralize carbonic acid excess. The low pH and increased carbonic acid concentration (pCO_2)* stimulate

---

* A decrease in alveolar ventilation if followed by an increase in arterial (or alveolar) partial pressure of CO_2.

the rate and depth of respirations to blow off excess carbon dioxide (hyperventilation). Through the kidneys, there is an increased formation of hydrogen ions in exchange for sodium, which is then reabsorbed with bicarbonate, thereby increasing available base. There is also increased formation of ammonia.

Shifts of electrolytes are not as marked in respiratory acidosis as in acidosis of metabolic origin. Often there are no intracellular changes. In severe, uncompensated respiratory acidosis, there may be shifts in extracellular and intracellular sodium, potassium, and chloride.

Changes in carbonic acid concentration instantaneously follow changes in alveolar ventilation, but secondary changes in whole blood buffers take more time. Therefore, a patient with acute respiratory acidosis in whom secondary metabolic changes have not occurred can promptly regain normal hydrogen ion control if alveolar ventilation is restored to normal.[3]

We see a patient who is dyspneic and hyperventilating at rest. There are often wheezing, tachycardia, and cyanosis. In the decompensated state there is shallow, gasping, rapid respiration with severe dyspnea and suprasternal retraction. Mental disorientation is often present.

Treatment of respiratory acidosis is very difficult because so frequently the patient is already a pulmonary cripple. The main goal is to improve the underlying pulmonary insufficiency through use of antibiotics, postural drainage, bronchodilators and detergents, inhalation therapy with nebulization, intermittent positive-pressure breathing, and the use of mechanical respirators if there is respiratory paralysis. Intubation and tracheostomy are often performed to establish an adequate airway.

A note of warning: there are pulmonary diseases such as emphysema in which the chronic anoxia serves as a respiratory stimulant. If this anoxia is taken away through use of oxygen, respirations may stop! It is not wise to slap an oxygen mask on every dyspneic patient!

Some patients are taught breathing exercises in which they learn to make expiration rather than inspiration the active phase of respiration. A recent advance in therapy has been the use of organic buffer compounds. One that has limited clinical use is trishydroxymethylaminomethane (THAM). It is used in severe cases and is administered intravenously at the rate of 300 ml per hour. Its therapeutic use awaits further clinical trial.

It is often a difficult task for the diagnostician to differentiate between the primary respiratory acidosis and the secondary respiratory alkalosis.

Metabolic Alkalosis

In any condition in which base bicarbonate or alkali reserve is increased with a concomitant decrease in hydrogen ion concentration, there is a metabolic alkalosis. For instance, in the vomiting patient large amounts of chloride are lost, leaving sodium unattached and available to combine with bicarbonate or change the carbonic acid-base bicarbonate ratio in favor of the latter. This same set of circumstances occurs when the nurse suctions the gastrointestinal tract vigorously without replacing electrolytes or gives the patient water to drink while an automatic suction machine is operating. Electrolytes are "washed out" with the water. If this chloride and potassium loss happens to be accompanied by acute stress, sodium is further retained and metabolic alkalosis is sure to occur. Uncorrected potassium loss because of lack of intake, suctioning, prolonged use of ACTH or cortisone, excessive parenteral administration of isotonic saline, or excessive administration of soluble alkaline powders leads to this condition.

This common disturbance of hydrogen ion control is chacterized by a decrease in hydrogen ion concentration (increased pH) and increased concentration of extracellular bicarbonate. The increase in bicarbonate may be due to administration of bicarbonate in excess, usually as sodium bicarbonate, to a deficit of body potassium, or to increased excretion of hydrogen in body secretions.

Buffer, pulmonary, and renal mechanisms attempt to compensate. Through buffer mechanisms, increased bicarbonate reacts with buffer acid salts, thereby decreasing extracellular bicarbonate concentration and increasing carbonic acid. Through pulmonary mechanisms there is a suppression of pulmonary ventilation with consequent increased carbonic acid concentration (pCO_2). The renal response is to conserve hydrogen and to excrete sodium and potassium with bicarbonate.

Thus, the compensatory mechanisms of metabolic alkalosis tend toward respiratory acidosis through hypoventilation and metabolic acidosis through buffer and renal compensation. Improper functioning of lungs or kidneys or deficiency of buffer systems will hinder the effect of the defensive mechanisms and result in uncompensated alkalosis with alkalemia.

The only reliable clinical sign associated with metabolic alkalosis is hypopnea.[3] This type of breathing is characterized by slow, shallow breathing. All thoracic movements are decreased, and periods of apnea may occur. Cyanosis may result when breathing becomes insufficient to meet oxygen needs. Other symptoms may include irregular pulse, renal insufficiency, paralytic ileus, muscle twitching with spasticity, and delirium. The behavioral changes begin insidiously and may be the first abnormality noted.[8] There is a change in personality. Patients who have been cooperative and alert become irascible, hypercritical, and belligerent. This is followed by dulling of the sensorium, drowsiness, and lethargy. Disorientation as to time and place may be present, accompanied by belligerent uncooperativeness.

SELF-INDUCED METABOLIC ALKALOSIS

In some patients with peptic ulcer taking large amounts of milk and readily absorbable alkali in the form of Sippy powders, sodium bicarbonate (baking soda), milk of magnesia, and calcium or magnesium carbonate, a moderately severe metabolic alkalosis may occur. An important element influencing the development of this syndrome is failure by the patient to precisely measure and limit the dose of the alkali to be consumed. Often, as in the case of sodium bicarbonate, the patient takes the substance without the advise of the physician in self-prescribed amounts. The substance promptly neutralizes gastric acid and makes the patient feel better initially, but then liberates carbon dioxide causing "carbon dioxide rebound" and an acidosis.

Unfortunately, the milk-alkali syndrome leading to an alkalosis occurs with greater frequency in older patients with hypertension and renal impairment, or in patients with potassium depletion. Early recognition of this condition is important because prolonged damage to the kidneys becomes irreversible. The first symptoms of milk-alkali syndrome are a distaste for milk, excessive dryness of the mouth and pharynx, and anorexia. Other early manifestations are general malaise, weakness, and lethargy. Polyuria is frequent. The important fact is that this syndrome is reversible if recognized and treated early. Antacids which are not absorbed from the intestinal tract, such as aluminum hydroxide gels, do not produce this sequence of events. Administration of intravenous sodium chloride and discontinuance of the alkali inducing the syndrome promptly correct the symptoms.

TREATMENT OF METABOLIC ALKALOSIS

The rationale of therapy is correction or amelioration of the primary disease or abnormality responsible for the alkalosis. Improvement of the compensatory mechanisms in order to allow for correction of the abnormal hydrogen ion concentration is the second goal of therapy.

When metabolic alkalosis is accompanied by the depletion of potassium stores, correction of the alkalosis will not occur until the potassium has been restored. If the alkalosis is the result of loss of chloride, 0.9 per cent ammonium chloride may be given intravenously. It should be injected slowly and is contraindicated in hepatic or renal failure. It is indicated in alkalosis due to use of mercurial diuretics in the edematous patient.

The ammonium ion is toxic when administered above the optimal rate.[9] The rate of flow is generally 2 to 3 ml per minute and is always less than 5 ml per minute for adults. If an excessive amount of ammonium chloride is administered, metabolic acidosis may result.

It should be noted that considerable difference of opinion exists relevant to the use of ammonium chloride; some authorities support its use, others state that it has limited usefulness. Isotonic sodium chloride is used in the treatment of extracellular chloride deficit.

Respiratory Alkalosis

In any condition in which there is hyperventilation not primarily resulting from an interference with pulmonary gaseous exchange, respiratory alkalosis may occur. Carbon dioxide is excreted at a faster-than-normal rate, and there is a resulting deficit of carbonic acid. We see a carbonic acid–base bicarbonate ratio of 1:40, which when partly compensated becomes 1:30, still with an increase in the bicarbonate radical. There is a lowered carbon dioxide combining power even though there is still an alkalosis.

Respiratory alkalosis is always due to central respiratory stimulation and hyperventilation. It is seen most frequently in the hyperventilation syndrome that accompanies hysteria and anxiety reactions. The syndrome may be self-induced and is often the aftermath of prolonged or strenuous exercise. Other conditions often producing respiratory alkalosis are fever, central nervous diseases such as meningitis, encephalitis, and intracranial surgery, and anoxia at high altitudes.

Buffer, pulmonary, and renal mechanisms function to compensate for the added bicarbonate. Through buffer mechanisms there is an increased rate of production of organic acids, which are made available to react with the excess bicarbonate ion. This tends toward restoration of the carbonic acid–base bicarbonate ratio of 1:20, and the pH is maintained at a normal value. Through pulmonary mechanisms there is depression or cessation of respiration, which compensates for the decreased carbonic acid. This lasts until sufficient carbon dioxide levels are reached in the blood to again stimulate respiration. Through renal mechanisms bicarbonate excretion is accelerated and hydrogen excretion is retarded.

The treatment, again, aims at striking the cause of the hyperventilation. Often, rebreathing carbon dioxide in a paper bag helps when the cause is hysteria. Of course, helping the patient dissipate anxiety is vital.

Confusion is inherent in the understanding of acidosis and alkalosis. Clinical signs may be absent or not easily detected. Various combinations of imbalance may be present in the same patient at the same time. Clinical signs of the metabolic and respiratory types of acidosis and alkalosis do not differ greatly. Laboratory tests combined with expert physical appraisal help in making an accurate diagnosis.

Emphasis for Nursing Practice

OBSERVATION OF BREATHING PATTERN

In any patient in whom an uncompensated acidosis or alkalosis exists or is a possibility, a most important nursing responsibility is the observation of depth as well as rate of respiration. If hyperpnea has been present and then has lessened, this is an indication that the acidosis is more severe; returning hyperpnea is an indication of improvement. The characteristic sign of hypopnea is the shallowness of respiration accompanied by limited chest movement. It is deplorable that observation of vital signs is so frequently delegated to ancillary personnel. Not only must the signs be observed, but the nurse must be able to compare these at varying intervals and then record and report vital changes. She must be aware of impending shock.

OBSERVATION OF BEHAVIORAL CHANGES

A number of mental and nervous signs may be present in acid-base imbalance, especially in alkalosis, due to hypoxia. These symptoms may be the initial cue to a change in the patient's condition. They include emotional lability, inability to concentrate, errors in judgment, tremors, mental confusion, and inordinate belligerence. It is so important for the nurse to actually pay attention to the patient's plea that he "just doesn't feel right!"

OBSERVATION AND MANIPULATION OF EQUIPMENT USED IN THERAPY

The nurse must always be aware of the hazards when patients are fed by vein. Rate of the drops per minute must be timed at several intervals because change in position alters the flow of solution. The nurse must be aware of the possibility of air embolus if bottles are left to empty and then are not shut off. She must check the patient's arm for possible infiltration. Many solutions cause caustic reaction if allowed to perfuse through the vein. The role of the nurse in parenteral administration is covered more thoroughly in related chapters.

The nurse must understand and know how to use positive-pressure breathing and nebulization apparatus. Although the manufacturers of these machines issue detailed operating instructions, nurses should take the time to familiarize themselves with the apparatus before they have to use it quickly. This is an excellent area for in-service education. Part of the responsibility of inhalation therapists employed by most hospitals is instruction of personnel in the proper use of this equipment. Often inhalation therapists are on duty only during the day shift. A few salient points regarding intermittent positive-pressure apparatus will be outlined here:

1. It is important that the face mask fit properly and be held firmly on the patient's face to ensure leakproof contact with the skin. An ill-fitting mask held loosely by careless or inexperienced personnel with an excessive amount of gas leaking out of the system will prevent the development within the lung of pressure high enough to operate the valve, it will not switch off, and the patient will receive continuous rather than intermittent positive pressure. The positive pressure can be applied during inspiration or during expiration.

2. The cooperative patient should be told that he is going to breath medicine and air, which will relieve his dyspnea and help him cough up mucus that is obstructing his air passages. If the patient is not accustomed to the machine, assure him that you will stay with him. Instruct the patient to remove the mask when he feels the urge to cough and to attempt to cough up as much mucus as possible.

3. The cooperative patient (one with whom it is possible to reason) should be ventilated for at least 15 minutes each time he receives the treatment. Encourage him to cough up secretion after each treatment. If the patient has the respirator attached to a tracheal tube, he will have to have continuous nebulization. Do not let the nebulizer dry out! As ventilization and nebulization liquefy secretions, they will rise continually into the upper air passages. Large mucus plugs will cause obstruction when this happens, and the respirator will switch on and off very rapidly. This is a warning that the respiratory passages and the tracheal tube require very thorough suctioning. It is wise not to let inexperienced or insecure personnel manage this suctioning because effective thorough suctioning is of vital importance to the patient. The importance of mouth care cannot be overemphasized; yet it is so frequently overlooked!

AWARENESS OF THE SIGNS OF
COMPLICATIONS OF THERAPY

Tetany may result from the treatment of metabolic acidosis with parenteral sodium bicarbonate. It may also be present in alkalosis and may result from prolonged hyperventilation. The clinical signs are tingling in the fingers and toes or about the legs, laryngeal stridor or "crowing" respiration, dyspnea and cyanosis, cramps of individual muscles as the tetany worsens, and finally tonic contractions of muscle groups. Calcium gluconate is sometimes administered concurrently with sodium bicarbonate to help prevent hypocalcemia.

These two substances are incompatible and should never be mixed. They will react to form calcium carbonate, which is insoluble and will precipitate. Calcium gluconate should never be given intramuscularly.

To avoid a toxic reaction caused by ammonium ions, ammonium should be administered at a rate not exceeding 400 ml per hour. Intravenous ammonium chloride is safe only when administered slowly.[10] Infusion bottles that contain this ion should be labeled, and the rate of flow should be clearly indicated. All personnel should be advised that the rate of flow may not be changed. If the physician does not specify rate of flow in the written orders, it is the responsibility of the nurse to obtain such written orders.

TEACHING THE PATIENT AND HIS FAMILY

Postural drainage is frequently prescribed for chronic pulmonary disease that is accompanied by a collection of secretions in the alveoli and respiratory bronchioles. There is a tendency by many patients to forego this treatment because the position is uncomfortable, the foul sputum that is raised leaves a very unpleasant taste in the mouth, and nausea and vomiting frequently accompany this procedure. The nurse should make sure the patient is adequately supported with his head and chest lower than his trunk to allow for gravity drainage. Stay with him! Time the treatment and gradually work up to a 20-minute treatment. Never use postural drainage for a longer period of time, and never after meals. Make sure the patient gets mouth care following the treatment.

The patient will often be sent home with specific instructions regarding kinds of foods and fluids to take. The physician may want to ensure an adequate quantity of liquid per day. The nurse must help in the instruction of patient and family. Nurses should advise against frequent self-medication with sodium bicarbonate, that old stand-by of the kitchen shelf, so frequently self-administered for "gas," upset stomach, heartburn, colds, or "acid stomach." The continued administration of sodium bicarbonate may result in chronic alkalosis.[11]

REFERENCES

1. STATLAND, H.: *Fluid and Electrolytes in Practice.* J. B. Lippincott, Philadelphia, 1957.

2. SCRIBNER, B., and BURNELL, J.: *Fluid and Electrolyte Balance*. University of Washington Press, Seattle, 1953.
3. BLAND, JOHN H.: *Clinical Metabolism of Body Water and Electrolytes*. W. B. Saunders, Philadelphia, 1963.
4. RAPPOPORT, S.; DODD, K.; CLARK, H.; and SYLLIM, I.: "Post Acidotic State of Infantile Diarrhea: Symptoms and Clinical Data," Amer J Dis Child, **73**:391, 1947.
5. FLETT, J.; PRATT, E.; and DARROW, D.: "Methods Used in Treatment of Diarrhea with Potassium and Sodium Salts," *Pediat*, **4**:604, 1949.
6. NAHAS, G.: "Use of Organic Carbon Dioxide Buffer in Vivo," *Science*, **129**:782, 1959.
7. MARIFREDI, P.; SIEKER, H.; SPOTO, A.; and SALTZMAN, H.: "Severe Carbon Dioxide Intoxication. Treatment with Organic Buffer (THAM)," *JAMA*, **173**:999, 1960.
8. GRACE, W.: *Practical Clinical Management of Electrolyte Disorders*. Appleton-Century-Crofts, New York, 1960.
9. KARR, N., and HENDRICKS, E.: "Toxicity of Intravenous Ammonium Compounds," *Amer J Med Sci*, **218**:302, 1949.
10. ZINTEL, H.; RHODES, J.; and RAVDIN, I.: "Use of Intravenous Ammonium-Chloride in the Treatment of Acidosis," *Surg*, **14**:728, 1943.
11. GOODMAN, L. S., and GILMAN, A. (eds.): *The Pharmacological Basis of Therapeutics*, 3rd ed. The Macmillan Company, New York, 1965.

ADDITIONAL READINGS

BEALE, H.; SCHILLER, I.; HALPERN, M.; FRANKLIN, W.; and LOWELL, F.: "Delirium and Coma Precipitated by Oxygen in Bronchial Asthma Complicated by Respiratory Acidosis," *New Eng J Med*, **344**:710, 1951.
BELAND, I.: *Clinical Nursing: Pathophysiological and Psychosocial Approaches*. The Macmillan Company, New York, 1965.
BROOKS, S.: *Basic Facts of Body Water and Ions*. Springer, New York, 1961.
DARROW, D.; DESILVA, M.; and STEVENSON, S.: "Production of Acidosis in Premature Infants by High Protein Milk," *J Pediat*, **27**:43, 1945.
DAVIDSON, I., and WELLS, B.: *Clinical Diagnosis by Laboratory Methods*. W. B. Saunders, Philadelphia, 1963.
DORMAN, P.; SULLIVAN, W.; and PITTS, R.: "The Renal Response to Acute Respiratory Acidosis," *J Clin Invest*, **33**:82, 1954.
ECKERIHOFF, J., and OECH, S.: "The Effect of Narcotics and Antagonists upon Respiration and Circulation in Man," *Clin Pharmacol Ther*, **1**:483, 1960.
ELKINGTON, J.: "Whole Body Buffers in the Regulation of Acid-Base Equilibrium," *Yale J Biol Med*, **29**:191, 1956.
GARB, S.: *Laboratory Tests in Common Use*. Springer, New York, 1958.
HARDY, J.: *Fluid Therapy*. Lea and Febiger, Philadelphia, 1954.
KIETEL, H.: *The Pathophysiology and Treatment of Body Fluid Disturbances*. Appleton-Century-Crofts, New York, 1962.

KOENIG, H., and KOENIG, R.: "Production of Acute Pulmonary Edema by Ammonium Salts," *Proc Soc Exp Biol Med*, **70**:375, 1949.

LIGHTWOOD, R.; PAYNE, W.; and BLOCK, J.: "Infantile Renal Acidosis," *Pediat*, **12**:628, 1953.

PETERS, J.; IANOWSKI, T.; GREENMAN, L.; WEIGARD, F.; GARVER, K.; MATEER, F.; and TARAIL, R.: "Acidifying and Nonacidifying Carboxylic Resin Mixtures Used Alone and with ACTH or Cortisone," *J Clin Invest*, **30**:1000, 1950.

RILEY, R.: "The Work of Breathing and Its Relation to Respiratory Acidosis," *Ann Intern Med*, **41**:172, 1954.

SHAFER, K.; SAWYER, J.; McCLUSKEY, A.; and BECK, E.: *Medical Surgical Nursing*. C. V. Mosby, St. Louis, 1964.

SLEISENGER, M., and FREEDBERG, A.: "Ammonium Chloride Acidosis: Report of Six Cases," *Circulation*, **7**:837, 1950.

SMITH, D., and GIPS, C.: *Care of the Adult Patient*. J. B. Lippincott, Philadelphia, 1963.

WINTERS, R.; WHITE, J.; HIGHES, M.; and ORDWAY, N.: "Disturbances of Acid-Base Equilibrium in Salicylate Intoxication," *Pediat*, **23**:620, 1959.

CHAPTER 5

Sodium and Water Imbalance

WHAT a dominant role sodium and water play in maintaining the isotonic balance between the intracellular and extracellular spaces! Increase or decrease the concentration of either sodium or water and the whole osmotic structure is altered. How remarkable it is, then, that in health each cell, though bathed in a solution primarily made up of salt water, maintains its own integrity!

In this chapter many new words will be introduced. Look at them closely and you will spot the symbol of the element in question. Hypo and hyper*na*tremia refer to decrease and increase in concentration of sodium in the blood. With rare exceptions, hyperosmolality (an increase in osmotic pressure or tonicity) and hypernatremia are seen together, and hypoosmolality (a decrease in osmotic pressure or tonicity) and hyponatremia are seen together. The terms "contraction" and "expansion" of fluid spaces are used to indicate, respectively, decrease and increase in fluid volume.

Our concern is primarily with change in extracellular water volume, either an excess or a deficit, and/or change in sodium content, either an excess or a deficit. Only occasionally do we see a simple loss or gain of either sodium or water. Usually, there is a variety of combinations of losses and gains, each having an ultimate effect on the other.

Water and Sodium

We can live without food for several weeks; we can live without water for only seven to ten days. There must be sufficient daily intake to allow for obligatory losses of about 1500 ml each day. There must also be ingestion of about 5 gm of sodium each day, although the adequately functioning kidney has the remarkable ability to conserve

63

sodium when intake is limited. The overused term "dehydration" has become a catchall to indicate a variety of losses and/or gains of both water and sodium salts. In this text the literal definition of dehydration, to mean an extracellular deficit of water and electrolytes in roughly the same proportion that they occur in the extracellular fluid, will be used. Overhydration, or volume excess, will be used to refer to an increase in extracellular water and electrolytes, again in roughly the same proportion that they occur in the extracellular fluid.

Physiological Occurrences in Water and Sodium Excess and Deficit

OSMOTIC CHANGES

Bland[1] has described volume excess and deficit in terms of tonicity, or the osmotic effect of constituents of one compartment on another. For example, an increase in the extracellular concentration of solute increases the tonicity of that fluid, which, because of the laws of osmosis, causes water to be drawn from the less concentrated intracellular spaces to the more concentrated extracellular spaces. Or if there is an extracellular water and sodium deficit with a loss of relatively more sodium than water, the tonicity of the extracellular spaces decreases and water moves from the extracellular spaces into the intracellular spaces. The terms "isotonic," "hypotonic," and "hypertonic" contraction and expansion are used by many experts to describe the various water and sodium imbalances. (See Fig. 2.)

HORMONAL CHANGES[2]

The "dehydration reaction" is stimulated by volume and osmotic changes in the vascular space. Aldosterone, known as the "electrolyte hormone," is secreted by the adrenals and causes retention of sodium and excretion of potassium. Retention of sodium conserves the water that would normally have been required to excrete the sodium. Potassium is excreted in greater quantities, possibly in an attempt to offset the increased tonicity of the extracellular sodium.

Antidiuretic hormone (ADH) is secreted by the posterior pituitary. It causes the kidney tubules to reabsorb more water. ADH is also secreted during severe stress and plays an important part in the overhydration seen following surgery.

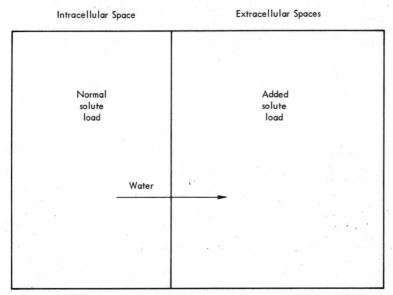

Intracellular Space   Extracellular Spaces

Normal   Added
solute   solute
load   load

Water

FIG. 2.   Osmotic changes caused by extracellular sodium excess.

There is increasing evidence that alcohol inhibits the release of ADH and causes diuresis. This tends to worsen an already water-depleted state. Alcohol also diminishes the normal thirst response. It inhibits release of ADH within 20 minutes after ingestion, and this effect may last as long as one month, with continued intake.[4]

Hormonal Response to Surgery

Surgery is a stressful experience and causes electrolyte and water changes that last from two to five days, depending on the extent of the surgery.[2] The hormone response is believed to be triggered by the contracted extracellular volume caused by accumulation of water and salts in and around the operative site. The "electrolyte hormone" aldosterone is secreted. Sodium retention and potassium loss follow. Studies reported by Marks et al.[3] indicate that it may be beneficial to plan for the decrease in volume by administering physiological saline preoperatively. This seems to cause a positive sodium-water balance by the third postoperative day. It is still possible to over-hydrate a patient during the first three postoperative days by allowing too large a volume of liquids either by vein or by mouth. (See Fig. 3.)

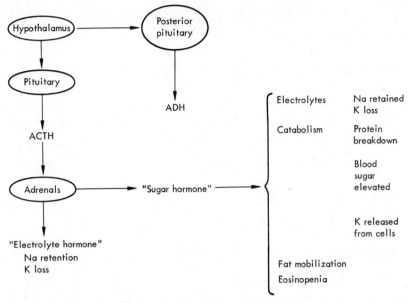

F<small>IG</small>. 3.   The stress reaction. (From H. Statland, *Fluid and Electrolytes in Practice*, 1957. Reprinted with the permission of J. B. Lippincott Company, Philadelphia.)

Some Combinations of Extracellular Volume and Sodium Changes

EXTRACELLULAR WATER DEFICIT PLUS SODIUM EXCESS

In this condition there is either a loss of water with a relative increase in sodium salt concentration or a genuine increase in sodium salt concentration with a decrease in water. We speak of sodium salts because sodium latches on to a variety of anions, along with chloride, in the body. Other descriptive terms in use for this imbalance include hypertonic contraction, primary dehydration, pure dehydration, water deficit, hypernatremia, solute loading dehydration, hypertonic dehydration, and sodium excess.

WHY DOES EXTRACELLULAR WATER DEFICIT PLUS SODIUM EXCESS OCCUR?

Thirst.   A simple failure to heed the thirst mechanism is the easiest road to this kind of deficit. Usually the volume and osmotic receptors in the blood vessels trigger the thirst center in the hypothalamus.[5] Most people respond by taking a drink. Some, however, are unable to drink. The semiconscious patient, the severely psychotic patient, and the apathetic geriatric patient may not heed the "get that drink of water" response. The hospitalized patient who does not care for "plain water" and who receives cold coffee and warm juice may acquire this deficit, as may the patient who cannot swallow without pain. Often this deficit goes unnoticed and progresses insidiously to dangerous physiological levels. We offer the infant water at periodic intervals because he cannot make his needs known through spoken language; it might be a good idea to offer our adult patients water at periodic intervals, too!

Impeded Kidney Conservation of Water. Sometimes the kidney fails to conserve water. In diabetes insipidus there appears to be lack of secretion of ADH, and large volumes of urine are excreted, leaving highly concentrated solute. The infant is particularly prone to loss of undiluted urine because his kidney is immature. He is also susceptible to large losses of electrolyte-free water through perspiration in extreme heat and through the stool.

Solute Loading. Increasing the tonicity of the extracellular space with added solute load is very common, especially in the hospitalized patient. A good example is the patient receiving nasogastric feedings of dextrose and amino acids, or concentrated milk drinks, without enough additional water to balance the added load. Infants fed undiluted cow's milk are overloaded. When the patient with a bleeding peptic ulcer is given milk and cream without water, there is absorption of partly digested blood and milk and cream with an increase in solute. In water loss caused by solute excess the patient voids large quantities of dilute urine. There is often a weight gain, rather than a loss, and this tends to fool the diagnostician.

Salt Poisoning. It is hard to believe that undiluted dry salt can be a culinary delight to young children. Yet a report by Calvin and Knepper[6] tells of two 14-month-old twins with severe extracellular water deficit and salt excess caused by ingestion of a box of common table salt! Evidently an older sibling left the salt in the crib as a plaything. As normal toddlers, the twins found it irresistible, and they ate it. Just about any item can be poisonous to curious toddlers. When they were admitted to the hospital they were very lethargic and their skin was hot and dry with decreased subcutaneous turgor.

Interestingly enough, they had neither diarrhea nor vomiting. This leads us to question the efficacy or safety of offering salt water to a person to make him vomit. Even in the face of severe hypernatremia,[7] the immature infant kidney excretes a dilute urine, so that the hypernatremia is, in effect, perpetuated and, if it continues, leads to interference with normal physiological function, possible brain damage, and death.

Water, Water, Everywhere. The Ancient Mariner had insight into a very practical solute problem when he said "water, water, everywhere, nor any drop to drink."[8] The ingestion of salt water, three times as salty as body fluid, increases the tonicity in the stomach. Water is drawn from the extracellular space into the stomach in an attempt to dilute it. When the pressure becomes unbearable, the stomach contents are vomited. Loss of fluid through vomiting further increases sodium concentration. The kidney is unable to keep up with this massive addition of solute.

EXTRACELLULAR WATER DEFICIT PLUS SODIUM DEFICIT

In this frequent condition there is a deficit of both sodium, with its anions, and water in roughly the same proportions as they exist in extracellular fluid. This is the literal definition of dehydration. It is encountered in any acute condition in which there is loss of water and electrolytes, such as severe vomiting.

SODIUM DEFICIT

In many instances there is a water and sodium deficit, but with relatively greater loss of sodium. The tonicity of the extracellular compartment is decreased, causing water to move out of the extracellular space and into the intracellular space. This leaves a contracted vascular and interstitial space and an expanded intracellular space. Other descriptive terms for this condition are hypotonic contraction, hypotonic dehydration, hyponatremic dehydration, hyponatremia, desalting water loss, sodium depletion, pure salt depletion, and low-salt syndrome.

WHY DOES SODIUM DEFICIT OCCUR?

Inadequate Sodium Ingestion Coupled with Use of Diuretic. In the normal diet salt, as sodium chloride, is replaced adequately. In a person with normally functioning kidneys a diet containing as little as 100 mg of sodium is sufficient; however, if the person should also be taking a diuretic, this deficit is frequently produced. Unaware that their weakness and lethargy are the result of the deficit, these people often become very depleted before they realize they should seek medical attention.

Loss Through Drainage. Whenever there are losses of gastro-intestinal body secretions, large amounts of sodium are lost. Vomiting, diarrhea, and fistulous drainage are frequent culprits. Often there is accumulation of sodium-containing fluids around the operative area following surgery. It is especially important for the surgeon to know if his patient has been on a salt-poor diet prior to the surgery.

Mechanically Induced Deficit. Body sodium is depleted when gastrointestinal contents are suctioned and the patient is offered sips of water or chips of ice while the suctioning is in progress. Sodium is "washed out" with the additional water. It is a good idea to use normal saline or a multiple electrolyte solution containing potassium to irrigate suction tubes, for this very reason.

Diluting Sodium Stores. In the absence of sweating a person needs 0.5 gm of sodium a day or less; however, on a very hot day we sweat profusely. Perspiration contains sodium. We lose sodium and water, but tend to replace only the water. This further dilutes the remaining sodium. It might be wise to salt the food on very hot days or to take one 0.5-gm tablet of sodium chloride with the water on a day when sweating is profuse.

The Lethal Tap Water Enema. Snively[8] tells of the "lethal tap water enema" given six times to a six-month-old infant by a tired, distraught mother to "make the child have a bowel movement." The baby became more and more fussy, began to draw her legs up in pain, and suddenly began to convulse. The tap water enema had "washed out" the salty intestinal fluid; the added enema water was absorbed into the extracellular spaces, diluting the remaining concentration of sodium. Fortunately, the child's life was saved by intravenous administration of sodium chloride solution.

Signs and Symptoms of Water and Sodium Deficit

Specific symptoms depend on the extent of the deficit. There can be losses of water ranging from 2 per cent of body weight, or 1 to 2 liters of water, all the way up to .8 per cent of body weight, or 5 to 10 liters of water.[2] There can also be salt losses ranging from 4000 to 10,000 ml of saline, or 0.5 to 1.25 gm sodium per kilogram body weight. In mild dehydration the only symptom present is thirst. On the other hand, a person experiencing severe dehydration might be comatose and on the brink of death. The laboratory findings are frequently deceptive. Concentration of sodium in the serum and urine may be increased, decreased, or unchanged in circumstances of either expansion or contraction of body volume.[1] Usually, dehydration is accompanied by hemoconcentration and oliguria and an elevated specific gravity of the urine.

The tools for bedside clinical assessment of body water and sodium stores are inadequate. Muldowney and Williams,[9] believing that alteration in total body water is reflected by changes in muscle content, report a method in which they have successfully analyzed lean muscle through biopsy procedure.

Along with laboratory findings, then, the physician pays particular attention to the physical findings and the fluid history. Such questions as "Has the patient vomited or had diarrhea, has he been eating and drinking in any special way, has he been on a sodium-restricted diet?" play a significant role in making the diagnosis. The signs and symptoms are classic. They are caused, generally, by a decrease in extracellular volume or a decrease in sodium salts.

From a decrease in circulating volume
Thirst
Loss of weight
Flushed, dry skin
Dry mouth and mucus membranes
Decrease in tissue turgor (when the skin is pinched it remains in the pinched position one-half minute or more)
Eyes appear sunken
Cold extremities
Drop in body temperature (there is an elevation when volume deficit progresses to very severe phases)
Generalized weakness
Drop in blood pressure
Tachycardia
Syncope with postural changes
Personality changes

Disorientation
Delirium
Coma

From a loss of sodium
Thirst is usually absent
Weakness
Apathy
Anorexia
Nausea
Vomiting
Feeling of faintness on standing
Muscle fatigue from usual exercise (i.e., it becomes a physical effort to shave or brush the hair)
Muscle cramps if water is suddenly ingested
Tremors
Muscle twitching and rigidity
Hyperirritability to stimuli
Dull headache, which becomes marked in the standing position
Mental confusion
Convulsions

Rationale of Treatment

The initial goal is to combat the shock by replacing lost fluids, volume for volume. Often, glucose is used with saline. It serves as a "protein sparer." It decreases the solute load for the kidneys by providing a substance to block the rapid breakdown of tissue protein.[1] If the loss involves gastrointestinal fluids, potassium is usually given. The physician attempts to treat the shock, stop further fluid loss, and give water and electrolytes to compensate for the loss.[5] He is careful to do this replacement gradually. The body may have become adjusted to the imbalance, and too rapid a correction would further disturb homeostasis. The nurse must be able to compare initial symptoms with changes in status following replacement therapy. She must also be familiar with signs and symptoms of too much potassium. (See Chap. 6.)

Water Excess in All Fluid Compartments

In this type of expansion there is a gain in volume of water in all the body fluid compartments. The water is able to permeate membranes to each of the major fluid compartments. There is no change in tonicity because the volume increase is equal in each compartment, and there is no electrolyte discrepancy. This type of expansion occurs when the kidneys can no longer handle the excess water. Other descriptive terms in use include hypotonic expansion and water intoxication.

Why Does Excess Volume Occur?

EXCESS ADH

In any stress situation, antidiuretic hormone is secreted, and there tends to be an increase in body water retention. The stress reaction can occur during severe fright, acute pain, and infections and after anesthesia, surgery, analgesia, and general trauma. The stress reaction is a common response to surgery, and it is very easy to cause a water excess in the postoperative patient by administering intravenous fluids and allowing drinking of water at the same time. Water excess occurs, also, in conditions such as Addison's disease and hypopituitarism.

DIMINISHED RENAL CIRCULATION

In numerous clinical conditions renal blood flow is diminished, and the kidneys cannot excrete sufficient water. This is particularly frequent in congestive heart failure and in cirrhosis of the liver. If water is "forced" as a diuretic in these conditions, the imbalance is worsened.

Signs and Symptoms of Water Excess

The symptoms depend on how quickly the water excess occurs. If the condition is acute, there is extreme progression of symptoms from muscle weakness, sleepiness, and loss of attention, to inco-ordination, changes in behavior, confusion, and delirium. If the water excess builds up slowly, the symptoms begin gradually. There are weight gain, weakness, apathy, sleepiness, anorexia, nausea, vomiting, marked salivation, and lacrimation, though there is no unusual sweating. The skin is warm, moist, and flushed. "Fingerprinting" occurs (when the finger is rolled over the sternum or tibia, the mark remains). There may be a moist, gurgling sound to the respirations. The tendon reflexes are diminished or absent, and there may be isolated muscle twitching. Laboratory studies indicate hemodilution. Voiding decreases.

Rationale of Treatment[5]

First, the water volume is reduced by withholding water for 24 hours. At least 1000 ml is then excreted through insensible water losses. Second, a hypertonic solution is administered. This enables the kidneys to excrete large volumes of water. The extra solute requires water for its excretion. We tend to forget that a patient can be seriously endangered from water excess. How important it is for the nurse to regulate the drops per minute of the intravenous feeding by counting for a full minute, at several intervals throughout the administration! A simple change in position can increase or decrease the drops per minute. It is also vital that the nurse understand just how much water the patient is permitted to take by mouth. Often this requires a call to the physician for verification. It is equally important for her to be fully aware of the signs of water excess, for her to realize that she can slow down the intravenous drops per minute or stop the solution completely, and for her to understand the importance of notifying the physician if she observes any of the above symptoms.

Extracellular Water Excess plus Sodium Excess

In water and sodium excess, or overhydration, there is an increase in the concentration and volume of the extracellular compartments, often because of the administration of hypertonic sodium chloride. With the increased tonicity of the extracellular space there is movement of water from the cells. This movement continues until the two compartments are again isotonic to each other, at which time there is excess of water and sodium in the extracellular spaces, but contraction of the intracellular space. We see symptoms of increased blood volume. There are a rise in blood pressure, rapid weight gain, dyspnea, hoarseness, edema, and a history of excess administration of saline solution.[1]

Edema

Edema is a condition in which the volume of the extracellular space outside the circulating intravascular compartment is increased. There is an increase in water volume and in sodium concentration, although the serum sodium is not elevated. Edema usually stems from a disruption in the pressure gradients within the capillaries. At the arteriole end of the capillary, the fluid pressure is greater than the osmotic pressure of the large protein molecules of blood, and fluid is pushed out into the tissue spaces. At the venule end, the osmotic pressure is less than the fluid pressure, and fluid is pushed back into the capillary. Both water and salts are retained. This fluid is not adequately used by the body to meet its requirements; an edematous patient, then, may actually be depleted of vital water and electrolytes available for use.

WHY DOES EDEMA OCCUR?

Damage to Capillary Membrane.   There are many instances in which capillary membranes are damaged and their permeability is increased. In the inflammatory response to mechanical injury, invasion by microorganisms, or any trauma, seepage of fluids through the capillary membrane occurs. This same response develops in sunburn, thermal or chemical burns, and allergic reactions; if too severe, it depletes the circulating plasma volume and causes shocklike symptoms.

Interference with Venous Flow with Alteration in Venous Pressure. In the horizontal position, the osmotic pull of plasma protein exceeds the venous hydrostatic pressure, and fluid re-enters the capillaries. In the standing position, however, the venous pressure rises. The massaging action of the muscles on the veins helps fluid to re-enter the capillaries, but if there is any interference with lymphatic drainage, fluid can accumulate in the tissue spaces. In the obese person, the massaging action of the muscles does not effect the desired result because fat pads interfere with their action. There is also an increase in venous hydrostatic pressure in persons with thrombophlebitis or varicose veins and in those wearing circular rubber garters.

Decrease in Plasma Protein.   When plasma protein decreases, the osmotic pull of fluid back into the capillary decreases, and tissue edema occurs. This is the reason we see the malnourished child with edema. This is also why we see edema of kidney disease with its loss of protein.

Edema occurs first in areas of low tissue tension, such as the eyelids and the genitalia. It is called "pitting" edema if the indentation following pressure with the finger remains. This indentation resembles a pitted area. Edema is called "dependent" when it occurs in areas in which gravity and position are the determining factors. Dependent edema occurs in the ankles when the person is standing, in the sacral area when he is sitting. Edema is called "refractory"[10] when diuresis remains inadequate following a full therapeutic regimen.

A person may be edematous and dehydrated at the same time. He may be edematous with a circulating salt deficiency. *Edema fluid cannot be used to meet obligatory requirements.*

MANAGEMENT OF EDEMA

The predisposing cause of the edema must be found and treated. When the illness improves, the edema improves as well. Next, salt is restricted to the amount that is normally lost daily, usually 2.0 gm or less each day. This allows for a gradual diuresis and avoidance of symptoms of low-salt syndrome. The amount of salt allowed varies with the condition of the patient. Water intake is restricted to the amount needed to meet obligatory losses. Often, intravenous salt-poor protein is administered to re-establish the capillary osmotic pull.

Cation Exchange Resins

These are insoluble, nonabsorbable synthetic polymers with chemical side chains that take up sodium and other cations in exchange for ammonium and hydrogen ions, which are absorbed by the intestine.[2] The remaining compound is eliminated through the bowel. These resins decrease the number of mercurial diuretics needed. They tend to be unpleasant to taste and may be constipating. Examples include Carbo-resin, Resodec, and Natrinil.

Diuretics

As reported by Gifford,[11] the new oral diuretics have replaced the weak and unpredictable xanthine and pyrimidine diuretics. The new diuretics are divided into sulfonamide compounds, such as chlorothiazide (Diuril), which block the reabsorption of sodium by acting as weak carbonic anhydrase inhibitors and steroidal spirolactones, such as spironolactone (Aldactone), which block the action of aldosterone on the kidney, thereby diminishing the exchange of potassium for sodium in the glomerular filtrate. This increases sodium excretion. These drugs have not replaced the potent parenterally administered mercurials; however, use of two potent but chemically different diuretics[10] in a "diuretic cocktail" seems to cause more effective diuresis. Often corticosteroids are used as one of the two cocktail ingredients, though the exact mechanics of how they produce diuresis is poorly understood.[10] Electrolyte and blood urea values should be determined at regular intervals during diuretic therapy. If the patient on diuretic therapy also experiences inadequate diet, vomiting, diarrhea, or loss of fluids through surgery, there may be a decrease in potassium (hypokalemia). In fact, even patients receiving a normally adequate diet when on therapy involving one of the thiazide diuretics often develop potassium deficit. Some drug companies include small amounts of potassium in the diuretic compounds; however, this amount is not enough to replace diuretic-induced loss.[11] Admonishing the patient to drink orange juice (0.45 gm K in 8 oz) or eat a banana (0.6 gm K in one banana) is equally inadequate. The patient who has a diuretic-induced potassium loss requires supplemental potassium intake, such as that available in Kaon Elixir or K-Lyte. Spironolactones are contraindicated if there is anuria or drug sensitivity. Sometimes a different but similar drug will be tried even with a history of drug sensitivity. Acidifying salts[2] such as ammonium chloride are frequently used because they supply excess anions for the excretion of cation. For the first four days of administration, body sodium is used for excretion of chloride. After the fourth day, however, ammonium (NH_4) has reached a point at which sodium is well protected. Ammonium chloride is not used for more than four days! It is usually administered for three days, then withheld for four days while the mercurials are given. The action of the mercurials is thus potentiated.

When diuretics are used, it is often difficult to estimate the total sodium loss. There is a definite possibility of salt deficit with water deficit or edema or with acid-base imbalance. When the edema is extremely resistant, peritoneal dialysis with solutions containing hypertonic glucose may be tried.[12]

The Patient with Congestive Heart Failure

Mrs. G. is a 50-year-old woman admitted to the hospital in moderate cardiac failure. She has had a history of heart disease for ten years, but only recently has experienced anorexia, weight gain, swollen ankles, and difficulty in "catching her breath" when doing her housework. The night before her admission she awakened at 3 A.M., sat bolt upright in bed, and appeared to be in a cold sweat. She was extremely dyspneic, coughed a good deal, and was very frightened.

Her initial orders read

ECG and prothrombin time stat
Oxygen tent p.r.n.
Morphine sulfate, 0.010 gm (gr 1/6) stat and q. 4h., p.r.n. for pain
Meralluride sodium (Mercuhydrin), 1 ml stat, I.M., and then O.D.
Spironolactone (Aldactone), 400 mg P.O., O.D.
Begin digitalization with digitalis, 1.5 gm in three divided doses day 1, then 0.1 gm O.D.
Thiamine chloride, 15 mg P.O., O.D.
Sodium-poor diet: 1.0 gm sodium O.D.
Fluids not to exceed 2000 ml O.D.
Record fluid intake and output
Complete bed rest
Semirecumbent position
Weigh daily

Here is a look at the sequence of events[13] that led up to this congestive heart failure. The two major precursors to all the symptoms were decreased cardiac output with inadequate oxygenation of the tissues and an elevated venous pressure with backup of fluids in the lung and right side of the heart. With the decreased cardiac output there were decreased renal blood flow and glomerular filtration rate, causing an increase in renal reabsorption of sodium. With the elevated venous pressure there was seepage of water and electrolytes from the vascular space into the tissue space. The blood volume was decreased and probably caused the secretion of aldosterone, which further increased the retention of sodium. Along with this, there was congestion in the liver with impairment of the usual aldosterone breakdown in that organ. The end result for Mrs. G. was generalized edema. There was pulmonary edema as a result of the pulmonary vascular bed receiving more blood from the right ventricle than the left could accommodate and remove.[14]

RATIONALE OF THERAPY

The main goals are to rest the heart by decreasing its work load and to decrease the extracellular fluid (edema).

REST THE HEART

Rest and activity orders vary. The physician weighs the advantage of decreased circulation against the possibility of formation of clots because of the sluggish circulation.[15] It is the responsibility of the nurse to understand the orders adequately and then to fulfill them by making purposeful nursing judgment. For instance, the physician may order complete bed rest. This indicates use of the bedpan. The nurse can choose the type of pan (i.e., the pediatric bedpan versus the adult-size pan); she can also observe the patient's reaction to the use of the bedpan and may suggest the use of a bedside commode to the physician if the pan causes great anxiety. The attitude of the nurse in fulfilling these mother-surrogate tasks for a dependent patient is empathized by the patient. If the patient becomes anxious, hostile, fearful, or angry, this increases the work load of the heart. It is up to the nurse to make judgments concerning the emotional response of the patient to her care. Morphine, by depressing the central nervous system, allays Mrs. G.'s anxiety and helps her to rest. Digitalis slows the heart and strengthens its contraction. Its action is potentiated by the diuretics. A general text in medical-surgical nursing discusses methods of resting the heart thoroughly.

REDUCING THE EDEMA

Winters and Gilmer[15] have summarized the purpose of diuresis as follows: "Diuresis, by reducing edema, relieves the severity of the dyspnea and this allays apprehension; the reduced dependent edema decreases the effort required for body movements, reducing the demands on the heart for oxygen."

The combined use of a mercurial diuretic and an aldosterone antagonist causes rapid diuresis. Too rapid a decrease in extracellular fluid might lead to low-sodium syndrome; the nurse must be alerted to possible symptoms such as weakness, nausea, vomiting, apathy, and dull headache. Aldactone causes potassium retention. The nurse must watch for weakness of the muscles, listlessness, cold extremities, etc. The rate of diuresis must be followed closely, by weighing the patient at the same time, on the same scale, and in the same clothes, every day. The preferred time is in the morning before breakfast and after the patient has emptied her bladder.

A truly accurate intake and output record is obtained only if the nurse and the patient work together. The patient is taught to jot down all liquids ingested, including liquid foods such as Jello and ice cream. The nurse makes a periodic check of this list, converts the amounts to milliliters, and records them.

Skin covering edematous tissue is poorly nourished and is likely to break down. The nurse encourages the patient to turn frequently and to move in bed. She takes the patient's limbs through a range of motion to increase circulation and decrease the chance of phlebothrombosis. She gently massages reddened areas with an emollient cream, paying particular attention to areas where the weight is borne (e.g., coccyx) and areas where the bony prominences are close to the skin, (e.g., shoulders).

The semirecumbent position helps decrease venous return to the heart and lungs and thereby diminishes pulmonary edema. In this position, the liver is less likely to press on the diaphragm, and this helps decrease the dyspnea.

The nurse plays an important teacher role regarding the sodium-poor diet. She reinforces the teaching of the physician and the hospital dietitian. Because she is with the patient for longer periods of time, she is able to ascertain just what the previous food habits were and how much of the presented dietary information was actually understood. Many nutritionists ask the patient to write a dietary diary of foods they normally ate throughout a usual day and then try to manipulate the sodium-poor diet around the patient's usual food habits. The following foods are common sources of salt.[16]

Salt. Medicines containing sodium; celery and garlic salts.
Bread, crackers, pancakes, salt-containing ready-to-serve cereals, cakes, spaghetti, macaroni.
Milk. Use Lonolac by Mead Johnson Laboratories or low-sodium milk by Walker-Gordon. Cheese, salt butter, margarine, sour cream.
Smoked and salted cured meats and salted fish, shellfish, ham, bacon, herring.

Bouillon and meat extracts used in soup. Beer. Pepsi-Cola.
Canned vegetables and soups. Any food with sodium benzoate added as
a preservative.
Spices. Dried fruits.
Pretzels, popcorn, potato chips, etc.
Beets, celery, kale, Lima beans, sauerkraut, spinach.

Commercial salt substitutes are available, though many patients
find them bitter and find that they leave an aftertaste. Diasal (KCl
with a trace of glutamic acid) is an example of a salt substitute.

When the daily sodium is decreased, water in amounts up to
3000 ml seems to further increase the diuresis. Care would have to be
taken, though, to prevent overloading the circulatory systems in
some patients.

General Implications for Nursing the Patient with a Sodium-Water Imbalance

OBSERVATION

Astute observation followed by knowledgeable action is one of the
most important factors in nursing the patient with dehydration or
overhydration. Using most of her senses to make the observation
(she sees the physical state; smells the breath; feels the skin; hears
the respiratory sounds), the nurse gets a clue as to his condition.
She then attempts to validate her tentative guess by instituting
further measures. For instance, a patient who is very weak and has
hot, dry skin may be dehydrated. He may also have a drop in blood
pressure from the decrease in circulating volume. The nurse takes
his blood pressure and then compares the results with prior readings.
She now has substantial proof that the patient may be dehydrated.
It is not enough to chart this information; she must make the physician aware of the patient's condition and carry out measures to
alleviate it, within the framework of written medical orders. No
symptom, objective or subjective, is too small for notice. The symptom may be the precursor to a change in condition. It may give the
physician the clue he needs to make an accurate diagnosis.

MOTHER-SURROGATE (SUBSTITUTE) MINISTRATIONS

Meeting the patient's basic needs adequately, and with a willing
attitude, is of utmost importance. The bedpan should be offered

periodically and its contents noted even in the absence of an intake-and-output order. The nurse should be able to report and record the status of urinary output.

An aesthetically acceptable supply of drinking water should be available. How often we "pour what's there" regardless of how long it has been standing there or how lipstick-stained the plastic carafe cover is! Some hospitals supply paper cups with the plastic pitcher, ensuring a clean receptacle with each drink.

The nurse must be aware of the amount of food the patient eats. Anorexia and fluid imbalances often go hand in hand. If a patient has poor appetite, thiamine and other vitamins are usually supplied. Instruction as to the type of diet comes throughout the patient's hospital stay and may be followed up by visits from a visiting nurse in the home. Referrals are made by the physician, but the actual mechanics involved in making the referral can be handled by the nurse.

How important the bath is! The gentle massage to the body so vitally aids the circulation to the often poorly nourished skin. This massage not only helps to prevent decubitus ulcers, but relaxes the patient and often takes the place of a tranquilizer!

Encouraging the patient to move, to change position, and to exercise his limbs (actively or passively) is vital to the prevention of circulatory stasis and phlebothrombosis.

RECORD OF INTAKE AND OUTPUT

The nurse is responsible for the accurate recording of fluid intake and output. Usually the physician requests a 24-hour record. It is a good idea to record eight-hour totals and a final 24-hour total. Van Pelt[17] suggests recording the three subtotals in red for clarification. The intake-and-output sheet should be at the patient's bedside, where it is seen easily and where it serves as a reminder to patient and nurse. Use of a sheet attached to a clipboard and left on the bedside stand has proved successful. A description of containers in use at a particular hospital and their volume content should be available. An example might be a chart[17] containing a description of the container (paper drinking cup), the fluid level or average portion (center line of blue trim), serving use (water with medications), and amount (60 ml). If an intravenous infusion is running when it is time to record an eight-hour total, the amount already absorbed is listed for that shift; the amount still in the infusion bottle is listed

in the space for the next shift. The combined 24-hour total of intake
and output is recorded on the graphic sheet of the patient's permanent chart.

INTERPRETATION OF ORDERS

Is the nurse quite sure of the physician's intention when she reads
"fluids ad lib"? Can the patient have more than 3000 ml? Up to
3000 ml? Should the fluids be plain tap water or should the nurse
encourage the patient to drink more physiological beverages such as
broth? Should salt be added to fruit juices? If the nurse is caring for
a second-day postoperative patient who is receiving 1000 ml glucose
in water by vein and is taking water by mouth, how much can she
allow him to take? Is she aware of the symptoms of overhydration
so frequently seen the first three days after surgery? Does she relate
anuria to possible overhydration and bring this to the physician's
attention; is there an order for daily intravenous infusions?

Effect of Drugs. Is the nurse aware that the action of digitalis is
potentiated by the potent diuretics? Does she realize that a patient
may be sensitive to the mercury in the mercurial diuretics and might
develop an allergic response to them (urticaria, nausea, vomiting,
dermatitis, suppression of white blood cell formation, fever)? Is the
nurse aware of the drugs that cause potassium retention? Can she
spot beginning symptoms of salt depletion?

SPECIAL THERAPEUTIC MEASURES

When pulmonary edema is severe, special measures are taken to
give the patient a measure of lifesaving relief. With production of a
stasis of blood in the veins, about 1000 ml less is transported to the
heart and lungs. Rubber-tube tourniquets (see Fig. 4) can be used;
they are tightened sufficiently to cause venous congestion without
obliterating the arterial pulse. Sphygmomanometer cuffs, if available,
are more accurate. They are inflated to a point slightly above the
level of the diastolic pressure.[14] The tourniquets are left on three of
the four limbs for no more than 15 minutes each limb. Using a
counterclockwise schedule, one tourniquet is removed every five
minutes and is applied to the unbound limb. It is important for the
patient to understand the purpose of the procedure and to realize
that the congested extremities will appear blue. One nurse should be

A. 10:00 A.M. Apply tourniquets to three limbs.

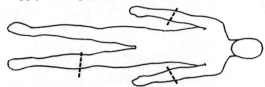

B. 10:05 A.M. Remove tourniquet from left leg and place on right leg.

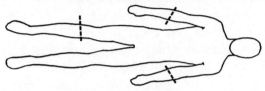

C. 10:10 A.M. Remove tourniquet from left arm and apply to left leg.

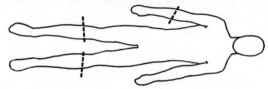

D. 10:15 A.M. Remove tourniquet from right arm and apply to left arm.

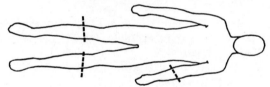

E. 10:20 A.M. Remove tourniquet from right leg and apply to right arm.

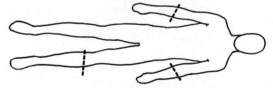

FIG. 4.   Rotating tourniquet schedule.

responsible for the procedure. She can map out a schedule and adhere to it rigidly.

Phlebotomy. This procedure, also called venesection, is used only if rotating tourniquets fail. With a standard blood donor set, 350 to

1000 ml of blood is removed from a vein. This instantly reduces the circulating blood volume and causes almost immediate relief of dyspnea, cyanosis, and systemic and hepatic engorgement.[16] It, too, is often a lifesaving process.

Paracentesis. In this procedure fluid is removed from a body cavity. Abdominal paracentesis is performed for ascites. The bedpan is offered before the paracentesis to lessen the chance of rupturing the bladder. The skin is anesthetized, a small incision is made, and a 4- or 5-inch trocar and cannula is inserted. After fluid begins to flow, a tube is attached and placed in a receptacle on the floor. The fluid flows by gravity. A sitting position best suits gravity drainage from the abdominal cavity. If the high-low bed, rather than a straight-backed chair, is used, care must be taken to make sure the collecting receptacle is not too far from the place of insertion. The pressure would be too great, and the elimination of fluid would be too fast. Shock might follow.

REFERENCES

1. BLAND, J.: *Clinical Metabolism of Body Water and Electrolytes.* W. B. Saunders, Philadelphia, 1963.
2. STATLAND, H.: *Fluid and Electrolytes in Practice.* J. B. Lippincott, Philadelphia, 1957.
3. MARKS, L.; GIBSON, R.; and OYAMA, H.: "Effect of Preoperative Isotonic Expansion of Extracellular Fluid Volume on Postoperative Renal Na Excretion," *Surgery,* **54**:456, 1963.
4. ROBERTS, K.: "Mechanisms of Dehydration Following Alcohol Ingestion," *Arch Intern Med,* **112**:154, 1963.
5. GOLDBERGER, E.: *A Primer of Water, Electrolyte, and Acid-Base Syndromes.* Lea and Febiger, Philadelphia, 1959.
6. CALVIN, M., and KNEPPER, R.: "Hazards to Health, Salt Poisoning," *New Eng J Med,* **270**;625, 1964.
7. HARRISON, H., and FINBERG, L.: "Hypernatremic Dehydration," *Pediat Clin N Amer,* **11**:955, 1964.
8. SNIVELY, W.: *Sea Within.* J. B. Lippincott, Philadelphia, 1960.
9. MULDOWNEY, F., and WILLIAMS, R.: "Clinical Disturbances in Serum Na and K in Relation to Alteration in Total Exchangeable Na, Exchangeable K, and Total Body Water," *Amer J Med,* **35**:769, 1963.
10. SELLER, R.; FUCHS, M.; SWARTZ, C.; BREST, A.; and MOYER, J.: "Treatment of Edema by the Combined Administration of Chemically Different Diuretic Agents," *Amer J Cardiol,* **12**:828, 1963.
11. GIFFORD, R.: "The New Oral Diuretic Agents and Their Clinical Applications," *Postgrad Med,* **37**:65, 1965.

12. LEVINSKY, N.: "Management of Chronic Renal Failure," *New Eng J Med*, **271**:460, 1964.
13. DAVIS, J.: "Mechanisms of Salt and Water Retention in Congestive Heart Failure," *Amer J Med*, **24**:486, 1960.
14. BRUNNER, L.; EMERSON, C.; FERGUSON, L.; and SUDDARTH, D.: *Textbook of Medical Surgical Nursing*. J. B. Lippincott, Philadelphia, 1964.
15. WINTERS, M., and GILMER, L.: "The Nurse's Judgment and the Patient's Understanding," *Amer J Nurs*, **61**:50, 1961.
16. FRIEDBERG, C.: *Diseases of the Heart*. W. B. Saunders, Philadelphia, 1956.
17. VAN PELT, V.: "A New Fluid Intake and Output Record," *Amer J Nurs*, **61**:80, 1961.

ADDITIONAL READINGS

BARTTER, F.: "Hyper- and Hypo-osmolality Syndromes," *Amer J Cardiol*, **12**:650, 1963.
BELAND, I.: *Clinical Nursing: Pathophysiological and Psychosocial Approaches*. The Macmillan Company, New York, 1965.
BELL, N.; SCHEDL, H.; and BARTTER, F.: "An Explanation for Abnormal Water Retention and Hypoosmolality in Congestive Heart Failure," *Amer J Med*, **36**:351, 1964.
BEST, C., and TAYLOR, N.: *Physiological Basis of Medical Practice*. Williams and Wilkins, Baltimore, 1955.
FUERST, E., and WOLFF, L.: *Fundamentals of Nursing*. J. B. Lippincott, Philadelphia, 1956.
GANN, D., and WRIGHT, H.: "Augmentation of Na Excretion in Postoperative Patients by Expansion of the Extracellular Fluid Volume," *Surg Gynec Obstet*, **118**:1024, 1964.
GOLDBERG, M.: "Hyponatremia and the Inappropriate Secretion of Antidiuretic Hormone," *Amer J Med*, **35**:293, 1963.
HOBLITZELLE, L.: *Pharmacology Applied to Patient Care*. F. A. Davis, Philadelphia, 1965.
HOLMES, J.: "Hyponatremia and Its Treatment in the Hospitalized Patient," *Amer J Cardiol*, **12**:644, 1963.
MUSSER, R., and SHUBKAGEL, B. L.: *Pharmacology and Therapeutics*, 3rd ed. The Macmillan Company, New York, 1965.
SANDERS, L., and MELBY, J.: "Aldosterone and the Edema of Congestive Heart Failure," *Arch Intern Med*, **113**:331, 1964.
SNIVELY, W.: *Highroad to Understanding Body Fluid Disturbances*. Mead Johnson and Company, Evansville, Inc., 1965.

CHAPTER 6

Imbalance of Potassium, Magnesium, and Calcium

> Potassium is not only the Star of the cell, it is also a sort of physiologic Doctor Jekyll and Mr. Hyde. "When it is good it is very, very good; but when it is bad it is horrid." SNIVELY[1]

ALL electrolytes are functionally interdependent and interrelated. In order to achieve proper physiological action they must be present in the fluids of the body in proper ratio to each other. Therefore, when an imbalance of any one electrolyte occurs, there is a concomitant imbalance of others. For example, in diabetic acidosis a deficit in both sodium and potassium accompanies the accelerated hydrogen ion formation. Although each chapter deals specifically with the imbalances of a particular electrolyte, it should be remembered that no electrolyte is individually altered. Disturbances in a single component of body fluid, water or electrolytes, seldom, if ever, occur. Instead, imbalances are usually multiple and complicated, although the imbalance of one may dominate the clinical picture.

Definition of Terms

Hypokalemia: refers to a potassium deficit in plasma.
Hyperkalemia: refers to an excess of potassium in plasma.
Kaluresis: refers to increased urinary excretion of potassium.

Total Body Content, Distribution, and Normal Plasma Values

The average total body content of potassium is 3200 mEq for men and 2800 mEq for women. The bulk of potassium is almost totally intracellular (98 per cent).

The normal plasma potassium concentration ranges from 3.5 to 5.5 mEq per liter.

Determination of the cellular content of potassium is exceedingly difficult; therefore, cellular potassium content is inferred from its level in plasma. This level may not always give an accurate picture of the amount of potassium in cells; for example, in the presence of excess intracellular potassium, the serum potassium level may be within the normal range.

Potassium Deficit

As stated previously, the kidney does not have as elaborate and precise a mechanism for the renal conservation of potassium as has evolved for sodium conservation. Potassium will continue to be excreted in urine, even in the event of no potassium intake. This is why one develops a potassium deficit so quickly when there is no potassium intake.

HOW DOES HYPOKALEMIA OCCUR?

The two principal avenues of potassium loss are the gastrointestinal tract and urine. (See Table 5.)

Table 5

CAUSES OF POTASSIUM DEPLETION*

A. Deficient intake—as in prolonged parenteral feeding without added potassium
B. Gastrointestinal losses
    1. Vomiting
    2. Continuous gastrointestinal suction
    3. Fistulas—biliary, pancreatic, intestinal
    4. Fecal—ileostomy, diarrhea, ulcerative colitis, frequent self-medication with drastic purgatives, repeated enemas
C. Renal losses
    1. Secondary to tissue breakdown—acidosis, trauma, diabetic ketosis
    2. Hormonal—Cushing's syndrome, primary aldosteronism, adreno-corticosteroid therapy
    3. Primary renal disease—diuretic phase of acute renal failure, chronic pyelonephritis, renal tubular acidosis
    4. Diuretics—particularly thiazide derivatives

---

*Modified from Bland, John H., *Clinical Metabolism of Body Water and Electrolytes*. W. B. Saunders, Philadelphia, 1963. Reprinted with permission.

Deficient Intake of Potassium.   Many patients with medical or surgical disorders suffer some potassium depletion. One of the contributing factors to this may be deficient intake. In a study of potassium deficiency in 404 surgical patients[2] it was found that 160 had hypopotassemia on admission to the hospital.

The majority of the 160 patients with hypopotassemia previous to admission had little or no intake of food for several days prior to admission. In many of these patients the inadequate intake was accompanied by additional losses due to vomiting, diarrhea, gastrointestinal fistulas, or hemorrhage.

Patients who are treated with a prolonged parenteral fluid regime that does not include the addition of potassium salts and who have little or no intake by mouth are subject to potassium depletion. In the above-mentioned study 67 patients had hypokalemia after varying periods (four days to five weeks) of hospitalization. All these patients had been on potassium-free intravenous fluids since admission. Prolonged use of parenteral fluid is often necessary to provide nutrition and prevent hypohydration. Often these solutions contain inadequate or no potassium.

The average normal intake of dietary potassium is from 0.8 to 1.5 gm per day. There is no storage of potassium; instead, any excess over and above current needs is eliminated in the urine. When inadequate intake or severe dehydration occurs, there is cellular damage, with a resultant release of potassium from the cells. This potassium is excreted in the urine.

Table 6

AMOUNT AND CONCENTRATION OF SODIUM AND POTASSIUM
IN GASTROINTESTINAL FLUIDS IN 24 HOURS

Secretion	Amount, ml	Sodium, mEq/L	Potassium, mEq/L
Saliva	1500	9	25.8
Gastric juice	2500	20–120	5–25
Bile	500	120–160	3–12
Pancreatic juice	700	110–160	4–15
Intestinal juice	3000	110–165	15–70

Gastrointestinal Losses.   Loss of gastrointestinal secretions is the most common cause of clinical water and electrolyte problems.[3]

This can be readily understood when the amount and composition of these secretions are taken into consideration. According to Gamble,[4] approximately 8 liters of fluid passes back and forth across the gastrointestinal mucosa daily. Inasmuch as this fluid is derived from the extracellular compartment, sodium is the dominant cation; nevertheless, potassium is present at higher concentrations in all gastrointestinal secretions than in extracellular fluid.

Normally, these secretions perform their function in digestion and absorption and are almost entirely reabsorbed. Potassium is almost completely reabsorbed, as fecal elimination amounts to only about 10 mEq per day. In a healthy individual with an adequate potassium intake, daily requirements for this ion are met entirely by intestinal reabsorption. In contrast, a sick individual with inadequate intake and with sustained losses of these secretions may quickly develop a potassium deficit. Compounding this situation is the fact that, in spite of increased loss of this ion through the gastrointestinal tract and inadequate intake, the kidney continues to excrete potassium.

Probably the greatest threat is to the patient who has undergone extensive surgery, who is taking nothing by mouth, and who requires continual gastrointestinal suction. Nasogastric suction removes gastrointestinal secretions; so there is a minimal amount of reabsorption of water and electrolytes.

Patients who have frequent watery stools, as in ulcerative colitis, are likely to develop potassium deficiency. The stool potassium content may be as high as 50 to 100 mEq per day in such patients.[5] In addition to the frequent stools there is hypermotility of the intestinal tract, which does not allow adequate time for intestinal absorption. The chronic use of laxatives and enemas may have the same results.

Table 7
AVERAGE GASTROINTESTINAL VOLUME LOSS

Source	Average Volume of Loss, ml
Vomiting	200–6000
Gastric lavage with water	0–25000
Suction drainage, small bowel fistula	200–7000
Diarrhea	500–8000

A Patient with Sustained Loss of Gastrointestinal Secretions

Mr. Thompson, aged 34, underwent an emergency operation for a ruptured appendix, complicated by peritonitis. The postoperative orders included continuous gastrointestinal suction, nothing by mouth, and parenteral fluids. The patient developed a paralytic ileus on the morning of the second postoperative day. He continually complained of thirst and pleaded for water—"Please, nurse, just a sip of water." The nurse was aware that the order nothing by mouth included sucking on ice chips or rinsing the mouth with water. As the patient's pleas for water became more and more constant, adding to his restlessness, the nurse called the surgeon. She asked him if he would permit the patient to have ice made by freezing a multi-electrolyte solution. The surgeon agreed to this. The patient was given small pieces of this ice, and his thirst was assuaged. When the nurse carried out the procedure of irrigating the gastrointestinal tube, she used isotonic saline as the irrigating solution, being careful to measure the amount used and the amount returned. The amount of secretions removed by suction was accurately measured and recorded on each shift.

Only certain aspects of the above case have been presented in order to illustrate those aspects pertinent to the present discussion.

What is the knowledge on which the nurse's judgment, and hence her actions, were based? Extremely thirsty patients frequently swallow the ice offered to them to suck on or the water used to rinse the mouth. The danger of swallowing this water lies in the fact that water given during the application of gastrointestinal suction will promote excessive intestinal secretory activity and upset isotonicity. In addition to the increased secretion, electrolytes will be drawn into the lumen of the gut and sucked out through the tube with resulting increased loss of electrolytes. Ice made from an isotonic solution will not disturb isotonicity. The nurse also knew that gastrointestinal tube irrigation is a depleting procedure. Deficits of sodium, potassium, chloride, hydrogen, or bicarbonate vary with the site of withdrawal from the gastrointestinal tract. The use of water or glucose in irrigating the stomach causes withdrawal of sodium, potassium, chloride, and hydrogen from the body. Introducing such solutions into the stomach "washes out" electrolytes. This does not occur if isotonic saline is used as the irrigating solution. The farther the tube descends into the intestine, the more damaging water can be. Water introduced into the ileum not only promotes intestinal secretion with resulting loss of electrolytes, but damages the in- testinal mucosa as well.[3] Accurate measuring and recording of the amount of secretions removed by suctioning provide the physician with information important in determining the amount of parenteral fluids to administer.

Renal Losses

Renal losses of potassium occur more insidiously than do gastro- intestinal losses. In addition, the patient with kidney disease is frequently not as seriously ill and can take an adequate intake by mouth.

Normally, around 75 to 100 mEq of potassium is consumed in the daily diet, and this is the amount that must be excreted in order to maintain potassium balance—when the renal losses of this cation are in excess of the intake, a deficit occurs. The conditions leading to such a deficit are listed in Table 5. Most of the potassium that is filtered through the glomerulus is probably all reabsorbed in the proximal renal tubule. The potassium appearing in the urine is the result of secretion of this ion by the cells of the distal tubule. In order for this secretion of potassium to occur, sodium ions are necessary for exchange with potassium ions; that is, the sodium ions present in the tubular urine exchange with the potassium ions in the renal tubular cell. Potassium ions compete with hydrogen ions in this cationic exchange process. For example, when the rate of hy- drogen ion secretion is decreased, as in renal compensation for alkalosis, the renal tubular secretion of potassium is increased.

Hormonal Influences on Renal Potassium Loss

The mineralocorticoids of the adrenal cortex, e.g., aldosterone and desoxycorticosterone, increase reabsorption of sodium from the renal tubule, promote secretion of potassium into the urine, and influence the rate of sodium and potassium transport across cell membranes, promoting entry of sodium into cells and extrusion of potassium from them. Aldosterone is the most potent of the salt-retaining hormones. This mineralocorticoid controls salt and water metabolism. The factors controlling aldosterone secretion are the blood levels of sodium and potassium and the degree of hydration. Aldosterone secretion is increased when blood sodium is low, blood potassium is high, or the patient is dehydrated. The physiological effect of this is obvious. Sodium holds tenaciously to water through its effect on osmolarity; by promoting renal reabsorption of sodium, aldosterone permits conservation of body water. In addition, it helps to rid the body of potentially toxic potassium in the extracellular fluid.

Potassium deficit is likely to be encountered in situations in which excessive amounts of adrenocortical hormones are present—during the administration of exogenous hormones and in the presence of a hyperfunctioning adrenal cortex, as in Cushing's syndrome and aldosteronism. Aldosteronism occurs in primary and secondary forms. Primary aldosteronism is most frequently due to an aldosterone-producing adrenal tumor, which causes an excessive secretion of aldosterone. The symptoms include persistent hypertension and often low serum potassium. Treatment is surgical removal of the tumor or subtotal or total adrenalectomy. Secondary aldosteronism occurs when the stimulus for the production of aldosterone occurs. Such stimuli are low serum sodium, very low intake of sodium, high potassium intake, and high serum potassium. The treatment is an increased sodium and decreased potassium intake.

Currently, potassium depletion via the urine is frequently a complication of diuretic and antihypertensive therapy. This is particularly true in relation to the thiazide group of diuretics, e.g., Diuril and Hydrodiuril. These agents apparently favor increased potassium excretion by presenting a larger load of sodium to the distal tubule for ionic exchange. The propensity of these drugs to produce excessive losses of potassium is no greater than that of other diuretics, but the fact that they are administered over a longer period of time, particularly in hypertension, does not give the patient a drug-free interval in which to reconstruct his losses from normal intake.

The most notable undesirable side effect of these compounds is hypokalemia. The chronic use of these compounds can lead to some potassium depletion. Patients on low-sodium intake are more likely to develop hypokalemia than are those whose sodium intake is normal. Hyponatremia may also occur. These deficiencies can be prevented by careful observation of the patient, adequate dietary intake of potassium, and replacement therapy with a potassium salt supplement.

In an attempt to overcome the electrolyte imbalance that occurs with the thiazide diuretics, considerable work has been carried out in several laboratories to design drugs that could (1) antagonize the action of aldosterone or (2) block the secretion of this mineralocorticoid. The consequence of this would be sodium diuresis accompanied by water excretion. One such compound that has been used clinically is spironalactone (Aldactone). This compound prevents the sodium-retaining effect of aldosterone, causing increased excretion of sodium and water and retention of potassium. Aldosterone is secreted in large amounts during the use of thiazides. Spiralactones act as metabolic antagonists to aldosterone and appear to be effective diuretic agents if aldosterone excretion is increased.[6]

The administration of a combination of chlorothiazide and spiralactones appears to be an effective method of treating edema, since disturbance of potassium balance is less likely to occur than with use of other drugs alone.[7]

Another compound currently undergoing extensive clinical trials in the United States is triamterone. It is probably an aldosterone antagonist.[8] It produces sodium and chloride excretion and reduced potassium excretion. It is reported to act more rapidly and to be more potent than spironalactone.[8]

Digitalis Toxicity and Potassium

Potassium antagonizes the action of digitalis. When the serum potassium level is low, an ordinarily nontoxic dose of digitalis may be sufficient to cause symptoms and signs of digitalis intoxication. Digitalis acts on cardiac muscle to promote a potassium deficit and thereby achieves a more profound digitalis effect in a patient with low serum potassium. Patients who are treated with both digitalis and diuretics, especially the thiazides, are especially prone to the possibility of severe digitalis intoxication because of the diuretic-induced hypokalemia. This can be offset by the administration of potassium salts.

Clinical Signs and Symptoms of Hypokalemia

The majority of the clinical signs of potassium deficit are non-specific. They may be found in many severely ill patients without low serum potassium levels. Moreover, multiple disturbances of homeostasis nearly always accompany potassium deficiency and may obscure its effects.

Potassium deficit results in disturbances in cellular function and disturbances involving a number of organ systems. The clinical signs are related primarily to disturbances of function in the neuromuscular, gastrointestinal, and cardiovascular systems. Profound changes may occur in the acid-base content of body fluids.

The clinical signs include the following, according to the system involved:

Neuromuscular: apathy, depression, generalized muscular weakness that may (rarely) progress to paralysis of the extremities and respiratory muscles. Cyanosis may be the most striking sign in patients with marked hypokalemia.

Gastrointestinal: progressive anorexia, nausea, decreased intestinal motility with resulting distention and paralytic ileus.

Cardiovascular: irregular pulse, hypotension, cardiac arrhythmias.

Laboratory Aids to Diagnosis

1. Determination of serum potassium levels. A concentration below 3.7 mEq per liter is suggestive of potassium deficit, and 3.3 mEq per liter or less is diagnostic. It is possible to have a severe potassium deficit with a normal concentration of the ion in plasma; nevertheless, the serum potassium concentration is currently the best laboratory aid to diagnosis. It is of greatest value when the various clinical conditions from which the patient may be suffering are taken into consideration (for example, acidosis, alkalosis, vomiting, and diabetes) and when serial determinations are carried out. Use of the electrocardiograph can also make serum potassium levels more meaningful.
2. Other tests on serum that may aid in diagnosis and give clues as to cause and progress include the serum content of sodium chloride and

calcium and the carbon dioxide combining power. The rationale underlying the use of these tests is that many of the signs and symptoms
attributed to hypokalemia may be due to disturbances in the pH or
in the sodium, calcium, or chloride concentration of plasma.

3. A simple and dependable method of determining the cell content of
potassium is not available. Tests sometimes used to determine this
value are muscle biopsy and determination of the potassium content
in red blood cells.

4. Examination of 24-hour urine specimen for potassium content.

5. The electrocardiogram may be utilized to reflect a loss of extracellular
potassium. Changes in the electrocardiogram suggestive of hypokalemia
are ST segment depression, a prolonged QT interval, and the appearance of a U wave.

Rationale of Treatment

Successful treatment depends not only on replacement of losses,
but also on therapy of the underlying disorder.

Potassium replacement is best accomplished by the oral route,
usually in the form of a potassium salt given as a supplement to the
diet. The dose is 5 to 10 gm of potassium chloride per day. If gastric
irritation results, the dosage may be changed to 2 gm every four
hours. If the patient cannot take anything by mouth, potassium is
administered parenterally. Parenteral potassium is most commonly
indicated for the patient who is unable to eat and who is on parenteral maintenance. In fact, one of the more common causes of
hypokalemia has been an iatrogenic effect, i.e., the administration of
potassium-free parenteral fluids over a long period of time.[3] The
usual parenteral (adult) dose is 40 mEq of potassium per liter daily.
In cases of great need for potassium this dose may be doubled or
tripled. The rate of intravenous infusion of a solution containing
40 mEq of potassium per liter should not exceed 15 ml per minute.[9]
If higher concentrations of potassium are used, the infusion rate
should be proportionately reduced.

The patient who is receiving intravenous potassium therapy should
be watched carefully for signs of potassium intoxication. Potassium,
it must be remembered, is predominantly an intracellular ion. Most
of the potassium administered or ingested promptly enters the cells.
The ready uptake of the ion by the cell is of vital importance in that

the cell fluid provides a buffer that prevents accumulation of excessive amounts in the extracellular fluid. If this were not so, the parenteral or even the oral administration of potassium salts might result in toxic extracellular concentrations. Potassium is the most sensitive ion of the extracellular compartment. Only a few milliequivalents difference in either direction may place the patient in a precarious state. For this reason, Snively[1] refers to potassium as the Dr. Jekyll and Mr. Hyde of the body's electrolytes, quoting: "When it is good, it is very, very good; but when it is bad, it is horrid." It must be emphasized that the patient may succumb to potassium intoxication even though the total amount in the body remains the same, because the toxic and lethal effects of potassium are due to the extracellular concentration of the ion.

In order, therefore, to guard against an abnormal concentration of plasma potassium, the physician may follow the patient with frequent determination of the serum potassium level and with electrocardiograms. Some physicians monitor the patient who is receiving potassium salts by vein with the electrocardiograph and may stop the infusion at the first sign of peaking of the T waves.

The major contraindication to potassium therapy is oliguria or anuria, for normal kidney function is the key to safe potassium therapy.

The incidence of digitalis toxicity is increasing. Dietary restriction of salt, parenteral administration of mercurial diuretics, and, particularly, the widespread use of the thiazide diuretics are probably the most important factors responsible for this rising incidence of digitalis toxicity. To counteract this, the physician may order potassium salts either orally or intravenously. The usual oral dose is 3 to 5 gm of potassium chloride given in divided doses daily. The initial dose may be 5 gm of potassium chloride in cold fruit juice. If parenteral administration is necessary, 40 mEq (3.0 gm) in 500 ml of 5 per cent glucose in water is used. The total amount is given over a period of one or two hours.[10]

Implications for Nursing Practice

Hypokalemia is now known to be a common clinical problem. Many patients will have some degree of potassium deficit as a result of current modes of therapy. The plight of these patients is better appreciated when it is known that the mortality rate of these patients is 5 per cent greater than that of patients who are not hypokalemic.[11]

PREVENTION

Prevention of the hypokalemic state is of prime importance. The nurse who familiarizes herself with those clinical situations that predispose to hypokalemia and who observes the patient carefully for the clinical signs indicative of this state will play a major role in prevention. The following clinical problems may predispose the patient to a deficit in potassium: inadequate potassium intake; vomiting; diarrhea; fistulous drainage; prolonged suction of the gastrointestinal tract; pyloric stenosis; diabetic acidosis; therapy with the thiazide group of diuretics; corticosteroid therapy; primary aldosteronism; the healing phase of burns; treatment with potassium-free intravenous fluids; and the diuretic stage of acute renal failure.

The patient's history frequently offers clues that will enable the nurse and physician to obtain valuable information. Not infrequently patients or their families will reveal information to the nurse that may not have been related to others. With today's emphasis in professional schools of nursing on the development and refinement of interviewing skills, the nurse practitioner, so educated, is in a prime position to obtain valuable clinical data. The history taking should include inquiries into the patient's nutritional history—his eating habits and how these habits may have been changed by illness. What about fluid intake? What medications has the patient been taking? Has vomiting occurred? How much? For how long? How often? Has the patient had diarrhea? How many stools per day? What about urinary output? Has there been reduction in flow? When did the patient last void? (Even rough estimates have value because the duration and magnitude of the losses are most important.)

Behavioral changes often are indicative of an electrolyte imbalance. The nurse may be the first to observe these. In potassium deficit these changes are most likely to include general lethargy and lassitude, accompanied by depression.

GASTROINTESTINAL SUCTION

In regard to the patient who is on gastrointestinal suction, the important nursing considerations in addition to the over-all comfort of the patient include accurate measurement of the amount suctioned, use of proper technique in irrigation of the tube (see p. 91), and attention to the functioning of the apparatus. Naturally, it is the responsibility of the physician to order the discontinuation of the suction, but usually the sooner it can be discontinued, the better. After discontinuation, a prime nursing responsibility is attention to oral intake. Too much emphasis cannot be placed on how liquids or other foods are offered to these patients. Imagine yourself on gastrointestinal suction for five days. The nurse or nursing assistant brings in your first cup of tea. Would you not like it on a tray with a cover, hot, and in a teapot, the cup on a saucer, offered to you with consideration and solicitude, and with an offer of assistance in drinking it? Such an attitude at this time is beneficial in encouraging the patient to eat and drink.

NUTRITION AND POTASSIUM SUPPLEMENTATION

When dietary intake is adequate, potassium supplements are usually not needed unless there are chronic renal losses, or unless thiazide diuretics are being given. One of the puzzling facts related to potassium deficiency in man is the rapidity with which normal potassium plasma levels are reached once the stomach begins to empty properly.[2] Gastric emptying is dependent on eating an adequate diet, even when taken in small amounts. In American hospitals we are as dedicated to the service of "three squares" a day as we are at home. Too frequently, hospital personnel—medical, dietary, administrative, and nursing—neglect the fact that the sick person often cannot eat three meals a day, but will eat well-cooked, appetizing foods in smaller amounts, more frequently. The importance of what and how much the patient eats cannot be overemphasized. According to Mudge,[12] the best way to administer potassium is in the form of a beefsteak. Potassium chloride frequently causes gastrointestinal irritation. Elderly patients are particularly prone to this side effect. There are various well-tolerated, palatable potassium products available. One such product is K-Lyte, an effervescent tablet form of potassium containing no chloride. Patients should be directed to dissolve the tablet in 3 to 4 oz of water to prevent gastrointestinal injury associated with the oral ingestion of concentrated potassium salt preparations. Enteric-coated potassium chloride tablets may cause small bowel ulcerations. As recently as April,

1965, the Food and Drug Administration placed enteric-coated potassium tablets on the prescription list with the requirement that they bear new warnings. Uncoated tablets and liquid preparations were also placed on the prescription list and required to carry "full disclosure" labeling and instructions on dilution. The following warning was published in the *Federal Register* of April 14, 1965: "Warning—there have been several reports published and unpublished, concerning non-specific small-bowel lesions consisting of stenosis—with or without ulceration, associated with the administration of enteric-coated thiazides with potassium salts. These lesions may occur with enteric-coated potassium tablets alone or when they are used with non-enteric coated thiazides or certain other oral diuretics. These small-bowel lesions have caused obstruction, hemorrhage and perforation. Surgery was frequently required and deaths have occurred. . . . Therefore, coated potassium-containing formulations should be administered only when indicated and should be discontinued immediately if abdominal pain, distention, nausea, vomiting or gastrointestinal bleeding occur. Coated potassium tablets should be used only when adequate dietary supplementation is not practicable."[13]

Some diuretics cause the extra excretion of 4 to 8 gm of potassium a day, and this much extra must be ingested. It is not possible to get sufficient potassium through the diet, therefore, it must be provided by *both* dietary intake and a potassium supplement. Table 8 lists common foods and their potassium content. The sodium content, which is also listed, must be considered if the patient is on a sodium-restricted diet.

Another contraindication to the use of oral potassium salts in therapy is relevant to the patient with heart disease. Potassium salts by mouth may produce toxic effects in these patients even when urinary output is normal.[14]

INTRAVENOUS THERAPY

Patients who are on parenteral administration of potassium salts must be observed for signs of hyperkalemia. The physician may order monitoring of these patients with the electrocardiogram, as this instrument is sensitive to changes in serum electrolytes. The physician may also want repeated laboratory determinations of serum potassium.

The State of Disequilibrium

Table 8

SODIUM AND POTASSIUM CONTENT OF VARIOUS FOODSTUFFS*

Food	Sodium (mg/100 gm)	Potassium (mg/100 gm)
Apple (less skin)	0.1	68
Apple juice, bottled (sweet cider)	4	100
Asparagus tips	2	240
Avocado	2	340
Bacon, fried crisp	3200	450
Banana	0.1	400
Bean, green	0.8	300
Beef	53	380
Bouillon cube	27,000	1500
Cabbage	5	230
Cantaloupe	12	230
Carrot	31	410
Celery (stalks)	110	300
Cereal, wheat (Maltex)	4	250
Cereal, wheat (Pettijohn's)	2	380
Chicken breast	78	320
Coca-Cola	1	52
Cocoa, powder	55	3200
Coffee, roasted	2	1600
Date	0.9	790
Fruit cocktail (canned, in syrup)	9	160
Grapefruit	0.4	200
Grapefruit juice (unsweetened, canned)	0.4	150
Liver, calf	110	380
Macaroni	1	160
Milk, malted	440	720
Milk, whole	51	140
Mushroom	5	520
Pea	0.9	380
Peach	0.1	180
Peanut butter	120	820
Pear, Bartlett	2	100
Pineapple	0.3	210
Postum (cereal beverage), dry	36	1300

*Compiled FROM Mead Johnson and Company, Evansville, Ind. Reprinted with permission.

Table 8 (*Continued*)
SODIUM AND POTASSIUM CONTENT OF VARIOUS FOODSTUFFS (CON'T.)

Food	Sodium (mg/100 gm)	Potassium (mg/100 gm)
Potato, sweet, less skin	4	530
Prune, dried	5	600
Raisin, seedless	21	720
Rice, puffed	0.8	100
Spinach	190	790
Squash, acorn	0.3	260
Tomato	3	230
Turkey, breast	40	320
Wheat, puffed	3	340
Wheat, shredded	2	240
Wine, port	4	75
Yeast, brewers'	8.320	2000

All intravenous flasks containing potassium salts should be clearly labeled. The wise nurse will insist that the physician, in writing, prescribe the rate of flow, and this information should be imparted to all nursing personnel and included in the labeling of the bottle. Because the rate of flow is so important, it should be noted at frequent intervals, and this should be recorded.

Unfortunately, clinical manifestations of potassium excess may occur late and may appear only a short time before death.[15] Bradycardia may be the first sign of hyperkalemia. Other symptoms include paresthesias, which may be of the scalp, severe weakness, extreme restlessness, and cardiac arrhythmias.

Potassium is contraindicated in renal failure, and in fact, in renal failure potassium may be lethal. Therefore, urinary output is measured and recorded. Any reduction in output should be reported.

Potassium Excess

HOW DOES HYPERKALEMIA OCCUR?

Hyperkalemia most commonly occurs as a result of acute renal failure and adrenal insufficiency. It may develop as a result of the parenteral administration of potassium salts. In renal failure the

diseased nephrons are unable to manufacture urine from the glomerular filtrate, and this filtrate is reabsorbed back into blood, trans-
porting with it water, electrolytes, and nonvolatile products of
metabolism. As a result the patient becomes loaded with water and
death may result from pulmonary edema. The increased rate of
catabolism associated with renal shutdown leads to hyperkalemia,
which may cause cardiac arrest. The end products of catabolism,
which are acid in reaction and many of which are toxic to the body,
increase in concentration since they cannot be excreted and may
cause death from uremia.

Adrenocortical insufficiency is accompanied by a loss of the ability
to adjust to a low intake of sodium, so that sodium is lost in the
urine and potassium retained. Treatment is the administration of
exogenous adrenocortical hormone.

A Patient Who Developed Acute Renal Failure

Bill Smith was driving home from college on his spring vacation.
His roommate, Ken, accompanied him. The boys had about 1300
miles to drive, and they wanted to make the trip quickly in order to
have as much time at home as possible. They decided to drive
"straight through," stopping only to eat. One slept or dozed while
the other drove. Bill was driving at night, with Ken asleep on the
back seat. The highway was monotonous, there was little or no
traffic, and he began to get sleepy. He pulled off the road, walked
around a bit, and took coffee from the thermos. This served to
awaken him. He started off again, feeling invigorated. He drove on
through the night, mile after mile. It began to rain and he started the
windshield wipers; their monotonous motion and sound seemed to
hypnotize him and he again became very drowsy. He saw the lights
of a town not far ahead, and he decided to drive on, hoping he would
find an all-night diner. Without realizing it, he dozed and was
awakened by headlights; too late he noticed that he was on the
wrong side of the road. He quickly swerved to avoid hitting the
oncoming vehicle and crashed into a concrete bridge abutment.

When the ambulance brought him and Ken to the hospital, Bill
was unconscious, bleeding, and in shock. Ken was conscious, and a
preliminary examination revealed that he was not as seriously

injured as Bill. A unit of dextran was started, and a vasopressor agent administered, and Bill was taken to the operating room for suturing and cleaning of his wounds. Typing and cross matching were done, and 1 liter of blood was started through a large-bore needle. From the operating room Bill was moved to the intensive care unit. His orders consisted of the usual measures used to combat shock. At the time of transfer to the intensive care unit he was still unconscious and hypotensive. He was placed in Trendelenburg position, which helped to infuse him with a unit of his own blood, and oxygen by nasal catheter was given at 6 liters per minute. The nurse made sure that the oxygen was humidified. His hematocrit was watched closely, and he was observed for further bleeding. Intake and output were carefully measured and recorded. The physician ordered another unit of blood to be followed by a liter of 0.9 per cent saline. As a result of control of bleeding, replacement of blood, and other supportive measures his blood pressure began to rise and consciousness to return.

On the afternoon following the accident the patient was conscious and oriented, and he was no longer hypotensive. He received parenteral fluids according to the physician's determination of need for water, electrolytes, and calories and was allowed fluids by mouth. The nurses continued to very carefully measure and record his intake and output. He was observed for loss of fluid through excessive perspiration. On the third postshock day his fluid intake by mouth and vein for the day shift was 2500 ml, but his urine output was only 225 ml. The nurse notified the surgical resident. The nurse also observed that the patient was less alert. The resident ordered immediate BUN and serum potassium determinations. The BUN was 92 mg per cent. On the previous day it had been 40 mg per cent. The serum potassium had risen from 4.9 to 5.8 mEq. The patient was started on conservative treatment for renal failure in the oliguric phase. During this phase there is almost complete renal retention of all waste products, electrolytes, and fluid. The treatment and rationale are as follows:

FLUID INTAKE

For this patient the daily fluid intake was limited to 600 ml plus the fluid output of the preceding day (urine, vomitus, or other fluid loss). Bill Smith had no extrarenal losses of fluid. The 600-ml fluid intake represents the difference between the insensible fluid loss from lungs and skin (1000 ml) and the water formed by tissue catabolism (400 ml).

DAILY WEIGHT

This is ordered to provide a check on fluid therapy. Proper fluid intake will be reflected by an average weight loss of 0.5 to 1 pound per day (this figure represents the amount of endogenous fat and protein metabolically consumed). If the patient does not lose weight, this is an indication that his fluid intake needs further reduction or he may become overhydrated, which may result in fatal pulmonary edema.

LIMITATION OF PROTEIN CATABOLISM

The following diet was ordered for Bill.

Total caloric intake: 1000 per day
Diet to include only the following foods:
  Hypertonic glucose (50 per cent) flavored with lemon juice
  Frozen salt-free butter balls (15 gm) sweetened with sugar
  Ginger ale
  Sweetened tea
  Hard candies
  Fat emulsions, e.g., Lipomul (UpJohn)
  Butter soup (sugar, 150 gm; salt-free butter, 150 gm; flour, 20 gm; water, 300 ml; and coffee extract)

The extracellular accumulation of potassium and the fixed anions of uremia is a consequence of protein catabolism. Therefore, the patient with renal failure is frequently acidotic and hyperkalemic. The high-fat, high-carbohydrate diet ordered for this patient has as its goal the suppression of protein catabolism. The most important consideration in the diet is that the carbohydrate intake be kept up for the protein-sparing effect of carbohydrate. At least 100 gm of glucose is needed daily to spare protein, i.e., minimize its catabolism.

LABORATORY TESTS

The following laboratory tests were ordered:

Serum electrolytes twice daily
CO_2 combining power daily
BUN daily

Creatinine daily
Electrocardiogram daily
Hematocrit daily

Acute renal failure is characterized by a progressive elevation of those metabolic end products that depend on the kidney for excretion, and so they accumulate in blood. Frequent determination of these products is necessary in order to evaluate the clinical course of the patient and the effect of the therapeutic regime. Anemia is frequently associated with acute renal failure and in Bill's case was associated with the acute blood loss he sustained. Electrocardiograms are essential in determining the effect on the myocardium of the electrolyte disturbance, especially rising potassium.

TRANSFUSE WITH FRESH PACKED RED CELLS

Bill's hematocrit was only 22 per cent. Obviously he was in need of blood. Fresh packed red cells were administered rather than whole blood in order to reduce the danger of pulmonary edema. Banked blood is further contraindicated, for, owing to the lysis of red cells in banked blood, it has a high potassium content.

ACHROMYCIN (TETRACYCLINE), 100 mg EVERY 12 HOURS

Infections are a serious complication in acute renal failure. The majority of patients dying from posttraumatic renal insufficiency succumb to infection.[16] The patient we are considering here, Bill Smith, has posttraumatic renal insufficiency plus multiple superficial and deep lacerations. Therefore, a broad-spectrum antibiotic is administered prophylactically. In renal insufficiency, antibiotics are poorly excreted; so doses are usually small.

In spite of the good clinical management and nursing care Bill's clinical course continued to run downhill. His serum potassium rose to 7.2 mEq per liter and he was uremic. The physician decided that he was a candidate for hemodialysis by the artificial kidney. The doctor called the physician in charge of the renal team at the state university medical center. They agreed to accept Bill for dialysis, and preparations were immediately made to transport him there by air ambulance. In general there are three indications for artificial dialysis in renal insufficiency: potassium intoxication with a rising serum potassium, systematic uremia (stupor, vomiting, rising BUN, convulsions), and pulmonary edema. The artificial kidney is most valuable in treating hyperkalemia and uremia of posttraumatic renal insufficiency.[16] Our young patient, Bill, met the first two of these contingencies.

In the interim, Bill was no longer able to take food by mouth. He had vomited, but this apparently had been controlled with chlorpromazine. However, it was necessary to keep up his caloric and carbohydrate intake. The physician ordered the following intravenous fluid order: 500 ml of 40 per cent glucose containing 5 gm of calcium gluconate and 50 units of insulin to be given slowly.

The glucose and insulin facilitate a prompt shift of potassium from extracellular to intracellular fluids. This effect, however, is transient, lasting no more than 8 to 12 hours. To avoid venous thrombosis from such a concentrated solution of glucose, it is administered through a thin, polyethylene catheter threaded into a large vein. It should be administered slowly. Five hundred milliliters of 40 per cent glucose contains 200 gm, or 800 calories. Calcium has an antagonistic action to potassium on the myocardium.

Upon arrival at the university medical center Bill was taken immediately to the renal treatment center, where preparations for dialysis had been completed.

HEMODIALYSIS

Dialysis refers to the separation of the crystalloids and colloids by a semipermeable membrane such as cellophane. This membrane permits the passage of solutes of low molecular weight, viz., electrolytes, but does not permit the passage of colloids, viz., proteins, bacteria, and viruses.

The primary purpose of an artificial kidney is the elimination of retention products in the blood. The artificial kidney duplicates the function of the glomerulus and the renal tubule in that retention products are withdrawn from blood by filtration and dialysis through a semipermeable membrane. The patient's blood is on one side of the membrane and an electrolyte bath on the other side. The direction of the movement of crystalloids is dependent on the difference in their concentration on both sides of the membrane. Thus, the specific electrolyte concentration of the dialysate determines the final blood concentration of these substances. End products of protein metabolism, such as urea, creatinine, and uric acid, will pass from the patient's blood into the dialyzing solution, because the bath does not contain these substances. In the use of the artificial kidney for acute renal failure, the dialyzing fluid does not contain potassium and thus it is withdrawn from blood.

In order to maintain the patient's blood volume and at the same time fill the dialyzing membrane, about 1200 to 1500 ml of blood is used. To prevent the blood from clotting, heparin is added. Blood is withdrawn from the patient through a plastic cannula placed either in the radial artery or in the saphenous vein. Blood is returned to the patient through a second cannula through a vein, usually the brachial. When the concentration of metabolites and electrolytes in the dialysate approaches that of blood, the fluid is changed. The procedure is terminated when the blood constituents are restored to normal or near-normal levels. The duration is usually six hours. The usual response is a marked clearing of mental symptoms, return to consciousness in a previously unconscious patient, and relief of nausea and vomiting.

The team at this particular renal center comprised five members: two physicians, two nurses, and a specially trained assistant. The responsibility of one nurse was in relation to the equipment and the procedure, with the second nurse in direct care of the patient. The patient must be weighed accurately immediately prior to and after dialysis in order to determine the exact amount of water removed by the machine. This may vary from 0.5 to 7 lb, with an average of 4 lb in a six-hour dialysis. Vital signs are noted on arrival in the kidney laboratory, and observations are made and recorded of the mental status of the patient. Serial blood pressure determinations are taken before the patient is connected to the machine and, after connection, are taken continuously until the doctor requests that they be stopped. It is important that these pressures be taken as rapidly as possible and called out loud enough for all to hear. This is of prime importance because it is on the stability of the blood pressure that the physicians rely to regulate the flow of blood through the machine. After the blood pressure is stabilized, it is taken every 10 to 15 minutes. To lessen the patient's discomfort, the nurse directly concerned with the patient eases the patient's tedious position by raising or lowering the head of the bed, placing a small pillow in the hollow of the back, and rubbing this area. Mouth care is necessary and ice chips are allowed. The patient's general condition is observed and any change is reported to the physician.

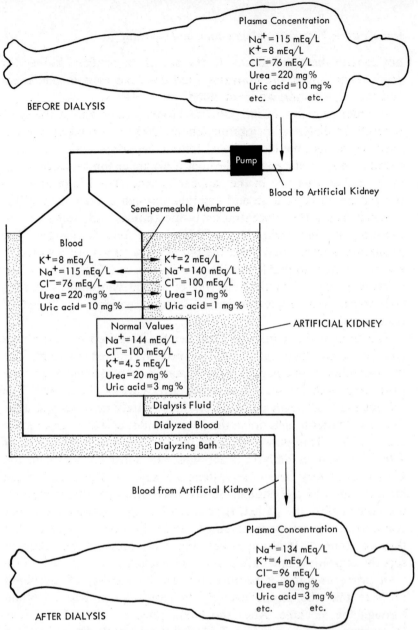

FIG. 5. Principle of artificial dialysis. In the patient with renal failure, there is usually an alteration of the electrolytes secondary to acidosis and failure of water and electrolyte homeostasis. At the same time, there is retention of organic acids and nitrogenous substances. As the blood is taken from the patient and pumped through the dialyzing membrane (which is submerged in the dialyzing fluid), the blood electrolytes and other substances tend to come in equilibrium with the concentration of these substances in the dialyzing bath. This is possible through the medium of the semipermeable membrane through which the blood is circulated. The blood is then returned to the patient. The process takes approximately six hours. (Redrawn with permission from G. Morris and J. Moyer: "Artificial Dialysis and the Treatment of Renal Failure," *Gen Pract*, **15**:103, 1957.)

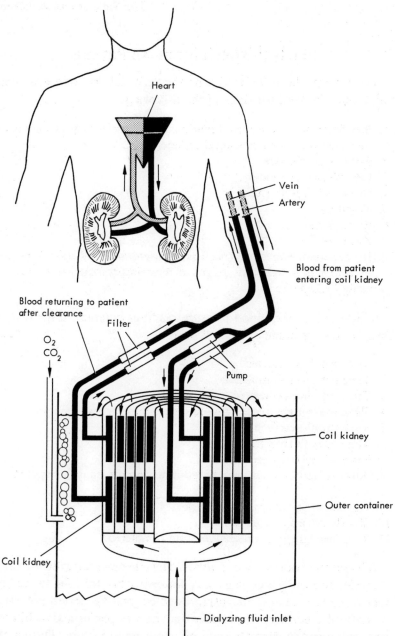

Heart

Vein

Artery

Blood from patient
entering coil kidney

Blood returning to patient
after clearance

Filter

O_2
CO_2

Pump

Coil kidney

Outer container

Coil kidney

Dialyzing fluid inlet

Fig. 6.   The Travenol Coil Kidney in relation to the patient and especially to the patient's kidney. It is evident from the diagram that the coil kidney is in parallel arrangement with the natural kidney, permitting full, simultaneous utilization of its remaining excretory capacity. (Redrawn with permission of Travenol Laboratories, Inc.)

Points to Watch for in All Patients

Any patient who is dialyzed is on the "critical" list, and a constant watch must be kept for signs of the following:

1. Bleeding due to repeated heparinization, particularly at cannulization sites and possibly femoral catheter sites.
2. Symptoms of shock.
3. Convulsions or tremors.
4. Changes in respiration.
5. Vomiting.
6. Restlessness.
7. Cyanosis.
8. In the patient who is suffering from an overdose of a dialyzable poison, or who is in uremic coma, signs of returning consciousness are especially looked for.

In addition to the blood pressure readings entered on the dialysis sheet, notes are made of the following:

1. Time cut-down started.
2. Time cut-down completed.
3. Time machine connected to the patient.
4. Time lost for any reason should the machine be switched off.
5. Time "run" resumed.
6. Time of bath change.
7. Time of heparin injections.
8. Any medications that may be given to combat nausea, hypotension, etc.
9. General observations and remarks.
10. Hourly record of vital signs.
11. Time machine disconnected and run completed.*

Bill Smith required five dialyses. His output gradually began to increase, and on the eleventh day following his transfer to the university medical center, his output doubled, and his serum potassium was 5.0 mEq per liter. No further dialysis was performed as Bill was now entering the diuretic state of acute renal failure. During this phase the regenerated tubules are lined with low cuboidal epithelial cells, which lack the ability to concentrate urea in urine, to conserve

* Maclean, Moira, "Role of the Nurse in Hemodialysis," Research Nurse, Renal Laboratory, Georgetown University Medical Center.

electrolytes, or to acidify urine. Actually, the glomerular filtrate is excreted almost unchanged.

The kidneys, though recovering, are functioning inefficiently and not as homeostatic organs. The patient at this time is usually in his most uremic state. Infection is the chief cause of death during the diuretic stage.[17] Convulsions and other signs and symptoms of severe uremia may appear during the first few days of diuresis. There may be excessive loss of electrolytes, and hypokalemia and hyponatremia may result. Usually fluids are not forced at this stage, as the fluid voided represents edema fluid. Supplemental potassium may be required. If the patient is able to take an adequate diet, he will not usually require supplemental potassium. The body weight should still be watched carefully. A return to a normal diet and early ambulation are important in this stage. Once diuresis is well established, no dietary restriction need be imposed. Most patients at this time will meet their nutritional requirements better if allowed foods of their own choice. Bill Smith's urine output rose to 5 liters per day. He was able to eat but did require supplemental intravenous potassium on two successive days because of a low serum potassium. After the peak output of 5 liters, his urine output gradually diminished until it approximated his intake. His weight remained stationary. He was alert, ambulating, and eating well. On the seventeenth day following his last dialysis he was discharged in care of his physician at home.

Other Treatments Used in Acute Renal Failure

PERITONEAL DIALYSIS

Peritoneal dialysis may be used instead of dialysis with the artificial kidney. It is one-sixth to one-tenth as efficient. In principle, the technique utilizes the large surface area of the peritoneal cavity as a dialyzing membrane. The composition of the dialysate is similar to that of blood minus the proteins and formed elements. Dialysis occurs only while the solution is in the peritoneal cavity. Usually within an hour, ionic equilibrium is reached between the dialysate and the patient's blood. The solution is allowed to drain out. The risk of infection is high, and paralytic ileus may result. This method of dialysis cannot be used if there has been a recent abdominal operation. If too much dialyzing fluid accumulates in the peritoneal cavity, this excess accumulation may enter the circulation, with

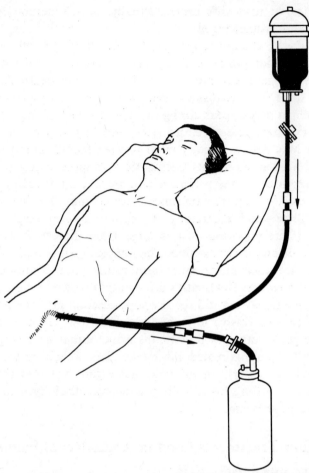

FIG. 7.   Method of intermittent peritoneal lavage for dialysis. The sterile lavage fluid is allowed to flow into the peritoneal cavity and remain there for two hours. The same bottle is then placed below the patient and drains out by gravity for a period of one hour. No more than 4,000 ml (4,000 cc) of dialyzing fluid should be allowed to accumulate in the peritoneal cavity (after Grollman). (Redrawn with permission from L. Bluemle: "Acute Renal Failure," *Gen Pract*, **41**:111, 1957.)

resultant pulmonary edema. In contrast, the artificial kidney has no contraindication other than uncontrolled hemorrhage.

CATION EXCHANGE RESINS

A potassium-binding resin may be given orally, in a dosage of 40 to 50 gm daily in divided doses. Because many patients usually cannot retain an orally administered resin, a 20 to 30 per cent suspension of the resin in tap water may be given rectally. This method is not considered very efficient. Resins are likely to cause fecal impaction and are usually given in conjunction with a cathartic.

OSMOTIC DIURETICS

Mannitol, an osmotic diuretic, may be given intravenously to maintain renal function during severe operations or immediately following severe injury.[18] It appears to have a preventive effect against the development of acute tubular necrosis leading to renal failure.

FUTURE DEVELOPMENTS

The day of the routine kidney transplant may not be far away. Successful transplants have been carried out in both identical and fraternal twins. The development of an implanted artificial kidney is not outside the realm of possibility.

Nursing Implications

The nursing care of the patient in acute renal failure is of the utmost importance. Prevention of complications is perhaps one of the most valuable nursing contributions because frequently the cause of death is attributed to the ensuing complications. Several medical writers[3, 16, 19] have attested to the importance of meticulous nursing care of these patients.

GENERAL NURSING CARE

Good oral hygiene, frequent turning, periodic deep breathing, forced coughing, tracheal aspiration, inhalations of cold mist, and early ambulation are mandatory prophylactic measures against pulmonary complications. In addition, proper positioning to allow maximal chest expansion is imperative.

PREVENTION OF INFECTION

As stated previously, infection is the major cause of death in patients with posttraumatic renal shutdown. All possible efforts should be directed toward prevention of infection. The patient should be in a single-unit room. Techniques of good medical asepsis should be adhered to. As much disposable equipment as is available should be utilized, including such items as surgical "prep" trays, needles and syringes, enema equipment, basins, and dressing trays. Personnel or visitors with any kind of infection should not be allowed near the patient. The changing of surgical dressings should be done only by the physician; this is not a nursing responsibility. Catheterization of the bladder should be avoided unless absolutely necessary because of the ever-present danger of introducing urinary tract infections. The physician may place the patient on isolation. As with any patient who must be isolated, the nurse must be aware of the feelings of loneliness and rejection that isolation frequently engenders.

NUTRITION AND FLUID INTAKE

The diet is usually very restricted and the fluid intake is limited. The allotted fluid intake should be divided over a 24-hour period. Strict control of the fluid intake is imperative. Unless this is done, the patient may die from overhydration. These patients usually suffer intensely from thirst. Frequent mouth care will help to alleviate this. Particular attention must be directed toward what the patients eat. The dietitian calculates the patient's diet according to the doctor's prescription. Any food or fluid not eaten by the patient should be returned to the dietary department to be recalculated, so that readjustment of the nutritional allotment can be made. As in any patient with a severe electrolyte imbalance, entire intake and output must be accurately measured. The patient's fluid intake usually includes 600 ml plus the previous day's output. This includes urine, vomitus, diarrhea stool, excessive perspiration, and any drainage. Fluids, given parenterally, usually consist of concentrated glucose solution. The vein into which the fluid is administered is to be watched for thrombosis.

PHYSICAL ACTIVITY

The nurse should have a clear and definite understanding of the amount of physical activity the patient may have. Usually, it is minimal in order to decrease the rate of metabolism. This requires that the nurses give complete care. Between the periods when the patient is turned, rubbed, and positioned, rest should be provided. This often constitutes a complex nursing problem and requires every skill of the nurse. These patients are often restless; yet because of the inability of the kidney to excrete, they may have no sedation, or sedation only in small doses. Therefore, every comfort measure must be utilized to provide rest.

During the diuretic phase, when the blood constituents have returned to normal, the patient should be more active and allowed ambulation.

DAILY WEIGHT

The daily weight is a guide to the amount of fluids the patient is to receive. On the therapeutic regime for patients in acute renal failure, the weight loss should be 0.5 to 1 lb daily. If the patient's weight remains stationary or if he is gaining, this means he is receiving too much fluid and is consequently overhydrated. The daily weight determination must be as accurate as possible. In order to ensure accuracy, the patient should be weighed on the same scales, after voiding, in the same amount of clothing, and at the same time. Weights usually show daily variations. For example, during a night's sleep the tendency is toward dehydration, with rehydration taking place during the day. If the patient cannot be weighed on a bedside scale, a stretcher scale may be used.

Hyperkalemia

Potassium intoxication represents the greatest threat in acute renal insufficiency. One of the most important signs to watch for is bradycardia. The following clinical signs may develop: absence of deep reflexes; sensations of tingling about the mouth, tongue, hands, and feet; paralysis of the extremities; and evidence of respiratory paralysis and cardiac arrhythmias. As cardiac arrest is always a possibility, the necessary equipment should be readily available. Survival of these patients depends not only on good medical management, but particularly on good nursing care throughout all phases of the disease.

Imbalances of Magnesium

Magnesium, like potassium, is predominantly an intracellular ion. The intracellular concentration of magnesium is 28 mEq per liter.

The extracellular concentration is 1.9 mEq per liter. Symptoms usually appear when the level reaches 1.5 mEq per liter and become severe at 1.25 mEq per liter. Magnesium is an essential element. Its presence is apparently essential to proper functioning of the neuromuscular system.

The great majority of orally ingested magnesium is excreted in feces. The fecal content varies with the magnesium intake; the amount that is absorbed is excreted in urine.

MAGNESIUM DEFICIENCY

Causes. Most commonly magnesium deficiency is seen in chronic alcoholism, with delirium tremens. Ordinarily, it is unusual to have an inadequate dietary intake of magnesium as it is present in all green plant foods, being the essential metal in chlorophyll. Chronic alcoholics usually have a grossly inadequate diet. Also, they frequently have diarrhea. Another frequent cause of magnesium deficiency is prolonged parenteral fluid therapy, which does not contain magnesium. Table 9 lists the principal causes of magnesium deficiency.

Table 9
PRINCIPAL CAUSES OF MAGNESIUM DEFICIENCY*

Chronic alcoholism
Prolonged parenteral fluid therapy without magnesium
Prolonged severe diarrhea
Vigorous diuresis
Renal disease before uremia
Acute pancreatitis
Primary aldosteronism
Diabetic acidosis
Hypoparathyroidism

*FROM Bland, John H., *Clinical Metabolism of Body Water and Electrolytes.* W. B. Saunders. Philadelphia, 1963. Reprinted with permission.

Clinical Signs. The clinical picture is principally characterized by neuromuscular and central nervous system hyperirritability. These findings are as follows:

1. A tremor is seen in most patients.
2. Aimless plucking at bedclothes.

 3. Athetoid and choreiform movements.
 4. Facial twitching and grimacing.
 5. Convulsions.
 6. Delirium.
 7. Confusion.
 8. Disorientation.
 9. Hallucinations—usually visual.
10. Delusions.

The tremors are characterized by irregularity. They wax and wane, sometimes disappearing for several hours and then suddenly reappearing. Although the hallucinations are usually visual, they may at times be auditory. The mental aberrations in these patients are striking.

Laboratory Aids to Diagnosis.

Determination of serum magnesium.
Twenty-four-hour urine for magnesium—the normal value is 4 to 20 mEq per day.

Treatment. Intravenous administration of magnesium quickly relieves the symptoms. The usual dose is 10 gm in 1000 ml of 5 per cent glucose. Proper precautions must be taken in order to make the intravenous administration safe. The infusion must be given slowly. A 1-liter infusion should be given over a one-and-one-half- to two-hour period. If magnesium sulfate is infused too rapidly, the patients complain of an intense, unbearable sensation of heat. Deep reflexes should be present at the start; if they become weak or disappear, the infusion should be discontinued. If a sharp drop in systolic pressure occurs, the infusion should be stopped. Injectable calcium gluconate should always be available. Calcium antagonizes the depressant action of magnelium. Magnesium therapy is contraindicated in patients with poor kidney function.

Magnesium sulfate may also be given intramuscularly. The injections are quite painful and should be made deep in the buttock. The initial dose is 8.0 gm daily in four divided doses, which after 48 hours is reduced to 4.0 gm daily.

Therapy is usually continued until the deficiency is corrected. In patients receiving prolonged parenteral fluid therapy, especially those on nasogastric suction, magnesium deficiency may be prevented by adding this ion to the electrolytes administered. When the patient is eating well, therapy may be discontinued.

MAGNESIUM EXCESS

The usual causes of this excess are renal insufficiency and severe dehydration. The signs and symptoms most commonly reported include respiratory embarrassment, lethargy, and coma.

The treatment is aimed at correction of the primary disorder, this consisting of the restoration of renal function and hydration. Dialysis may be indicated. All magnesium-containing compounds should be withheld. Ten per cent calcium gluconate is usually administered to offset the toxicity of the magnesium ion.

A Look at Calcium

As mentioned in Chapter 2, 99 per cent of the calcium in the body is located in the skeleton, while only 1 per cent is found in the soft tissues and extracellular spaces. Not all of the bone calcium is available for rapid ionization. The "structural" bone, made up of "old" highly mineralized, poorly hydrated cells, is fairly stable and serves primarily for bony support. It can be mobilized, slowly, by parathyroid action. The "metabolic" cells are less well mineralized, are well hydrated, and are quickly mobilized in response to serum calcium levels. Of the 1100 gm of calcium in bone, only 5 gm exists in readily usable form.[20] This ionizable calcium is in sufficient quantity to buffer decreases and increases in serum calcium levels and acts independently of parathyroid hormone.

Many factors affect the absorption and retention of calcium, although their interrelationships are not clearly understood. For instance, there exists a reciprocal relationship between the levels of calcium and phosphate in the blood.[21] An elevation of one accompanies a decrease in the other. In the presence of hypercalcemia there is hypophosphatemia, and vice versa. There must be adequate intake of calcium, phosphorus, and vitamin D for normal bone metabolism. This requirement is usually met in the American diet, rich in milk and milk products. An adult will be in "calcium equilibrium" when he ingests 10 mg calcium per kilogram of body weight, about 800 mg calcium per day, or the equivalent of two glasses of milk each day.[22] For adequate calcium metabolism there must be normal gastric acidity, to allow for absorption of soluble calcium salts, and a large enough intake to allow for precipitation in the intestines of 80 per cent of the calcium as insoluble calcium salts.[22]

Action of the Parathyroids

The two pair of parathyroid glands, embedded in and surrounding the thyroid, release their hormone (parathormone) in response to low serum calcium or high serum phosphate levels. The hormone, a protein substance, has as its main goal maintenance of the concentration of calcium ion activity in the plasma within narrow limits, despite wide fluctuations in calcium intake and excretion.[23] The hormone increases reabsorption of calcium in the kidney, resorption (lysis) in bone, and absorption in the gastrointestinal tract. When the serum level is re-established, the parathyroid secretion is automatically shut off.[23] The parathyroids evidently affect the rate at which these metabolic processes take place. If the glands are damaged, as is often the case during thyroid surgery,[20] calcium metabolism continues, but the serum calcium level is lower.[3]

The two chief theories regarding the manner in which parathormone increases serum calcium are, first, that it mobilizes calcium and phosphate from bone in response to serum level of calcium, and, second, that it acts primarily on phosphate. With increased phosphate excretion there is a concomitant decrease in calcium phosphate, and this, in turn, stimulates the mobilization of bone mineral.

Both the adrenal and parathyroid hormones affect calcium metabolism.[20] They are antagonistic to one another. The steroids tend to depress serum calcium, the parathyroids to increase it. If the steroids are administered to a patient, who unknowingly, has hypoparathyroidism, an acute hypocalcemic syndrome (tetany) may be precipitated.[20]

CALCITONIN

There is increasing evidence that the parathyroids produce not only the slower-acting hypercalcemic parathormone, but a more rapidly acting hypocalcemic hormone called "calcitonin."[24] This second hormone seems to be secreted in response to high serum calcium levels. Its specific function is the prevention of hypercalcemia caused by excess parathormone production. The action of calcitonin is lost when the parathyroids are removed.[24]

HYPERCALCEMIA

An excessive ingestion of calcium is not the cause of hypercalcemia. In the normal adult, calcium not needed for metabolism is excreted; however, excessive ingestion of calcium by a person with a condition that causes increased calcium absorption or decreased renal excretion may cause hypercalcemia, with vitamin D intoxication. This is seen in Paget's disease, osteoblastic metastatic disease, hyperparathyroidism, malignant metastases to bone, thyrotoxicosis, adrenal insufficiency, and prolonged excessive intake of milk with alkali (reversible).[22] Early laboratory tests show a fall in the concentration of plasma phosphate rather than an elevation of calcium.[23] Symptoms include nausea, anorexia, lethargy, polyuria, thirst, azotemia, and weight loss. If hypercalcemia is prolonged, regardless of the cause, there is impairment of renal concentrating ability and there may be vascular calcification.[22] The cause of the hypercalcemia must be located and treated. If the hypercalcemia is not of parathyroid origin, cortisone may be used to reduce serum calcium levels. There is some evidence that hyperventilation may cause hypercalcemia.[25]

HYPOCALCEMIA: TETANY

The patient who experiences fatigue, grimacing, muscular weakness, constipation, palpitations, and numbness of the extremities may be in a hypocalcemic state[20] and may show overt signs of tetany during a stress situation such as a high fever. There is abnormally increased reaction of motor and sensory nerves to stimuli (neuromuscular hyperirritability) with painful tonic spasms of groups of muscles or the entire body musculature.[26] Facial spasm produces stiffness and rigidity, with typical "tetany facies." The cardiac muscle is stimulated. There are carpopedal spasm and larynogspasm and paresthesias, frequently followed by convulsions.

Carpal spasm may be produced (Trousseau's phenomenon) as a diagnostic aid by inflating a manometer on the arm for 1 to 5 minutes. A positive reaction consists of production of typical contraction of the fingers and hand.

A positive Chvostek sign is also indicative of tetany. This is a facial nerve phenomenon in which there is momentary contraction of the lip, nose, or entire side of the face when areas of the face are tapped. A positive peroneal sign in which there are dorsal flexion and abduction of the foot when the peroneal nerve is tapped is also an indicator.

Hypocalcemia is seen in a number of conditions, including hypoparathyroidism, rickets, osteomalacia, chronic renal disease, and malabsorption syndrome. It is found in alkalosis because calcium and magnesium ions migrate to muscle cells, decreasing the amount of ionized calcium in the serum.[22] Pregnancy often causes symptomatic hypocalcemia.

Newborn babies, fed cow's milk, often have tetany during the first ten days of their lives. This may be because of the immaturity of their parathyroid glands and the relatively large phosphate load in cow's milk.[22]

Hypocalcemia can be corrected by administration of calcium salts by mouth (calcium chloride and lactate, 1 to 2 gm 4 × O.D., or gluconate 5 gm, 3 × O.D.), intramuscularly (calcium gluconate, 1 gm O.D.), or intravenously (calcium chloride, 5 to 20 ml of 5 per cent solution or gluconate, 1 gm O.D.). Calcium salts are given in conjunction with large doses of vitamin D, 50,000 to 400,000 U.S.P. units O.D. For maximum absorption, calcium salts should be given one half to three quarters of an hour before meals and at bedtime. The chloride, containing the largest quantity of calcium, is also the most irritating to the gastrointestinal tract. Calcium gluconate can be ingested over longer periods of time and is used most frequently.[26]

REFERENCES

Potassium

1. SNIVELY, W.: *Sea Within.* J. B. Lippincott, Philadelphia, 1960.
2. EVANS, E.: "Potassium Deficiency in Surgical Patients," *Ann Surg,* **131**:945, 1950.
3. BLAND, JOHN H.: *Clinical Metabolism of Body Water and Electrolytes.* W. B. Saunders, Philadelphia, 1963.
4. GAMBLE, J.: *Chemical Anatomy, Physiology and Pathology of Extracellular Fluid.* Harvard University Press, Cambridge, 1947.
5. KIETEL, H.: *The Pathophysiology and Treatment of Body Fluid Disturbances.* Appleton-Century-Crofts, New York, 1962.
6. TUBLIN, I., and BERMAN, L.: "Treatment of Edema with an Orally Administered Spironolactone," *JAMA,* **174**:7, 1960.
7. OGDEN, D.; SCHERR, L.; SPRITZ, N.; and RUBIN, A.: "Comparison of the Properties of Chlorothiazide, Spironolactone, and a Combination of Both as Diuretic Agents," *New Eng J Med,* **265**:358, 1961.

8. deStevens, G.: *Diuretics*. Academic Press, New York, 1963.

9. Goodman, L. S., and Gilman, A., (eds.): *The Pharmacological Basis of Therapeutics*, 3rd ed. The Macmillan Company, New York, 1965.

10. Spain, D.: *The Complications of Modern Medical Practices*. Grune and Stratton, New York, 1963.

11. Surawicz, B.; Braun, H.; Crum, W.; Kemp, R.; Wagner, S.; and Bellet, S.: "Clinical Manifestations of Hypopotassemia," *Amer J Med Sci*, **233**:603, 1957.

12. Mudge, G.: "Potassium Imbalance," *Bull NY Acad Med*, **29**:846, 1953.

13. Food and Drug Administration: "Potassium Salt Preparations Intended for Oral Ingestion by Man," *Federal Register*, April 14, 1965.

14. Brown, H.; Tanner, G.; and Hecht, H.: "The Effects of Potassium Salts in Subjects with Heart Disease," *J Lab Clin Med*, **37**:506, 1951.

15. Swonn, R., and Merrill, J.: "The Clinical Course of Acute Renal Failure," *Medicine*, **32**:215, 1953.

16. Morris, G., and Moyer, J.: "Artificial Dialysis and the Treatment of Renal Failure," *Gen Pract*, **15**:103, 1957.

17. Merrill, J., and Franklin, S.: "Acute Renal Failure," *New Eng J Med*, **262**:711, 1960.

18. Moore, A.: "Tris Buffer, Mannital and Low Viscous Dextran," *Surg Clin N Amer*, **43**:577, 1963.

19. Grace, W.: *Practical Clinical Management of Electrolyte Disorders*. Appleton-Century-Crofts, New York, 1960.

20. Kahn, A.; Snapper, I.; and Drucker, A.: "Corticosteroid Induced Tetany in Latent Hypoparathyroidism," *Arch Intern Med*, **114**:434, 1964.

21. Beland, I.: *Clinical Nursing: Pathophysiological and Psychosocial Approaches*. The Macmillan Company, New York, 1965.

22. Weisberg, H.: *Water, Electrolyte, and Acid-Base Balance*. Williams and Wilkins, Baltimore, 1962.

23. Rasmussen, H.: "Parathyroid Hormone-Nature and Mechanism of Action," *Amer J Med*, **30**:112, 1961.

24. Copp, D.; Cameron, E.; Cheney, B.; Davidson, A.; and Henze, K.: "Evidence for Calcitonin—A New Hormone from the Parathyroid that Lowers Blood Calcium," *Endocrinology*, **70**:638, 1963.

25. George, W. K.; George, W. D.; Smith, J.; Gordon, F.; Baird, E.; and Mills, G.: "Changes in Serum Calcium, Serum Phosphate, and Red Cell Phosphate During Hyperventilation," *New Eng J Med*, **270**:726, 1964.

26. Paschkis, K.; Rahoff, A.; and Cantarow, A.: *Clinical Endocrinology*. Paul B. Hoeber, New York, 1958.

ADDITIONAL READINGS

Potassium

Barry, K.: "Post-traumatic Renal Shutdown in Humans: Its Prevention and Treatment by the Intravenous Infusion of Mannital," *Milit Med*, **128**:224, 1963.

BLUEMLE, L.: "Acute Renal Failure," *Gen Pract*, **41**:111, 1957.
BOBA, A.; LANDMESSER, C.; and POWERS, S.: "Prophylactic Aspects of Post-traumatic and Postoperative Renal Failure," *New York J Med*, **63**:812, 1963.
BURNELL, M., and SCRIBNER, B.: "Serum Potassium Concentration as a Guide to Potassium Need," *JAMA*, **164**:959, 1957.
CORCORAN, A.: "Renal Failure," *Amer J Nurs*, **56**:768, 1956.
HAWK, P.; OSER, B. L.; and SUMMERSON, W. H.: *Practical Physiological Chemistry*, 13th ed. Blakiston Division, McGraw-Hill Book Company, New York, 1954.
LANS, H.; STEIN, I.; and MEYER, K.: "Diagnosis, Treatment and Prophylaxis of Potassium Deficiency in Surgical Patients," *Surg Gynec Obstet*, **95**:321, 1952.
LUBRAN, M., and McALLEN, P.: "Potassium Deficiency in Ulcerative Colitis," *Quart J Med*, **20**:221, 1951.
MACLEAN, M.; CREIGHTON, H.; and BERMAN, L.: "Hemodialysis and the Artificial Kidney," *Amer J Nurs*, **43**:1672, 1958.
MERRILL, J., and FRANKLIN, S.: "The Artificial Kidney," *Sci Amer*, **205**:56, 1961.
SINGER, M.; HOFF, R.; FISCH, S.; and DEGRAFF, A.: "Red Blood Cell Potassium," *JAMA*, **187**:34, 1964.
SNIVELY, W.: "Fluid Balance in Obstruction of the Large Intestine," *J Indiana Med Ass*, **53**:427, 1960.
SPENCER, R.: "Potassium Metabolism and Gastrointestinal Function: A Review," *Amer J Dig Dis*, **4**:145, 1959.
TESCHAN, P., and BAXTER, C.: "The Future of Hemodialysis in Military Medicine," *JAMA*, **166**:11, 1958.

Magnesium

FANKUSHEN, D.; RASKIN, D.; DIMICH, A.; and WALLACH, S.: "The Significance of Hypomagnesemia in Alcoholic Patients," *Amer J Med*, **37**:802, 1964.
FLINK, E.; STUTZMAN, F.; ANDERSON, A.; KONIG, T.; and FRASER, R.: "Magnesium Deficiency After Prolonged Parenteral Fluid Administration and After Chronic Alcoholism Complicated by Delirium Tremens," *J Lab Clin Med*, **43**:169, 1954.
GERST, P.; PORTER, M.; and FISHMAN, R.: "Symptomatic Magnesium Deficiency in Surgical Patients," *Ann Surg*, **159**:402, 1964.
PRITCHARD, J.: "The Use of Magnesium Ions in the Management of Eclamptogenic Toxemias," *Surg Gynec Obstet*, **100**:131, 1955.
SMITH, W.; HAMMERSTEIN, J.; and ELIEL, L.: "The Clinical Expression of Magnesium Deficiency," *JAMA*, **174**:77, 1960.
————: "Magnesium Deficiency in the Surgical Patient," *Amer J Cardiol*, **12**:667, 1963.
SUTER, C., and KINGMAN, W.: "Neurologic Disorders Linked to Magnesium Depletion," *Neurology*, **5**:691, 1955.
VALLEE, B.; WERCHER, W.; and ULMER, D.: "The Magnesium Deficiency Tetany Syndrome in Man," *New Eng J Med*, **262**:155, 1960.
WEISBERG, H.: *Water, Electrolyte and Acid-Base Balance*. Williams and Wilkins, Baltimore, 1962.

Calcium

FRAME, B.; FRUCHTMAN, M.; and SMITH, R.: "Chronic Hypocalcemia in a Patient with Parathyroid Clear Cell Hyperplasia," *New Eng J Med*, **267**:1112, 1962.

MUSSER, R., and SHUBKAGEL, B. L.: *Pharmacology and Therapeutics*, 3rd ed. The Macmillan Company, New York, 1965.

CHAPTER 7

Multiple Water and Electrolyte Problems

WE have discussed single-element imbalances for ease of presentation; however, an ill person frequently presents multiple water and electrolyte imbalances, often complicated by acidosis or alkalosis. These imbalances are usually categorized as "mixed excesses and depletions." The burned patient falls into this category.

The Burned Patient

THE STORY OF MRS. BROWN

It was a particularly harassing day for this 30-year-old mother of four children. She had been up with her youngest during the night, and by lunchtime the next day she was exhausted; her patience was worn thin. The children were hungry. A batch of French fried potatoes seemed like the perfect appeaser. The deep fat was set on the stove to heat. When one of her children happened to wander inquisitively toward the stove, she grabbed him and, in pulling him away from the danger, accidentally knocked the kettle of hot grease on herself. She ran screaming from the house, and a neighbor called the rescue squad.

She was taken to the burn unit of a general hospital. This is a self-contained area designated specifically for the care of victims of burns. It houses all the specialized equipment required, including such items as a tub with thermostatic temperature control and water agitator, circular electric beds and Stryker frames, an air-purifying system, a mechanical respirator, and an artificial kidney. Other equipment kept on hand includes intravenous infusion setups, a variety of intravenous fluids, cut-down and tracheostomy sets, and prepackaged bundles of sterile linen. The unit is located near the surgical suite and is staffed by a highly trained group known as "the burn team."

An immediate initial appraisal of the extent of the injury was made. Mrs. Brown was estimated to have second-degree burns of the right side of her face and neck and third-degree burns of part of her right arm and the anterior portion of her chest. In Figure 8 heavier shadowing indicates third-degree burns and lighter shadowing indicates second-degree burns;[1] the estimated area of burn was 20 per cent.

It is difficult to make an accurate initial estimate because of the similarity in appearance between second- and third-degree burns. Many differentiating tests have been devised, though none has been proved infallible. Some authorities maintain that a hair lifts out of its follicle easily in third-degree burns; some state that capillary function is destroyed in third-degree burns and that, by injection of dyes such as Patent Blue V (similar to gentian violet) into the blood stream, second- and third-degree burns can be differentiated. In third-degree burns the skin is nonviable and there is no alteration in color following injection, whereas in second-degree burns the skin is viable and turns a distinct blue following injection with the dye.[2] Still other authorities test for the degree of anesthesia in the burned part.

A specimen of blood was obtained immediately for baseline studies of hematocrit and electrolytes. A Foley catheter was inserted for hourly urine measurements, and an indwelling polyethylene tube was inserted into the left femoral vein under local anesthesia. Five hundred milliliters of plasma was started. A tracheostomy set was available in case subsequent edema of the face and neck blocked the trachea. Mrs. Brown weighed 130 lb (59 kg).

Our patient was fortunate in that she had no pre-existing renal or cardiac disease to complicate the already serious picture. The fact that the total area of body involvement was not over 20 per cent indicated that, barring complications, she would probably survive. More than 30 per cent involvement is usually fatal.[3] The patient's age, too, was in her favor. Patients under 50 respond better to therapy than patients over 50. Five thousand units of tetanus antitoxin was administered, as was 600,000 units of procaine penicillin.

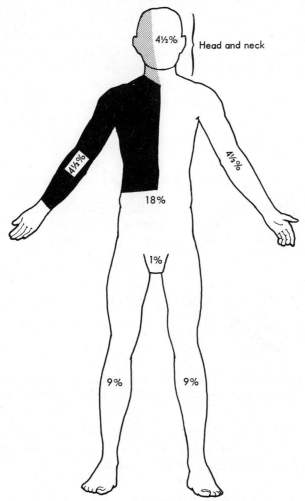

FIG. 8.   Twenty per cent body burns.

Mrs. Brown was taken to the operating room, where the burn was washed gently with a pHisoHex and sterile water solution; all loose epidermis was removed, and blisters were gently broken. Open-air treatment was selected in lieu of covering the burns with dressings. If the burn encircled parts of the body and the patient was forced to lie on them, dressings would be used to encourage crust formation. Morphine sulfate, 15 mg (gr¼), was administered for pain.

There is some evidence[4] that ice water is an effective therapeutic measure in burns of less than 20 per cent. There is an immediate alleviation of pain and an apparent decrease in the usual burn sequelae. The cooling is continued, sometimes for several hours, until the pain does not recur when the burned part is withdrawn from the cold bath. Ice-cold towels are used if it is not feasible to immerse the part. Evidently the time factor plays an important part in the effectiveness of the treatment. The sooner the immersion, the better the result.

What Are Burns?

Burns are tissue injuries caused by thermal, electrical, or chemical agents, and by most forms of radiant energy.[3] They are classified according to depth and percentage of body involvement.

Depth[5] of Burns

First-degree burns are superficial, partial-thickness injuries involving only the epidermis. There are redness (erythema), edema, and pain.

Second-degree burns involve the epidermis and the dermis without destroying the dermis. The skin is reddened and painful. There are vesicles (blisters) with oozing.

Third-degree burns involve the epidermis and dermis, with destruction of both. The skin is charred or pearly white, and dry. Because of nerve destruction, there is no pain.

Percentage of Body Involvement

The well-known "rule of nines"[1] is used to determine percentage of area involved. For adults, the areas are divided as shown in Figure 9. For children, different percentages are allowed for various parts of the body. For instance,[6] the head and neck of a one-year-old are allotted 19 per cent. This amount decreases by 1 per cent with each year of age, until it reaches the 9 per cent of the adult. The lower extremity of the one-year-old child makes up only 13 per cent of the surface area, but this increases five tenths of a per cent per

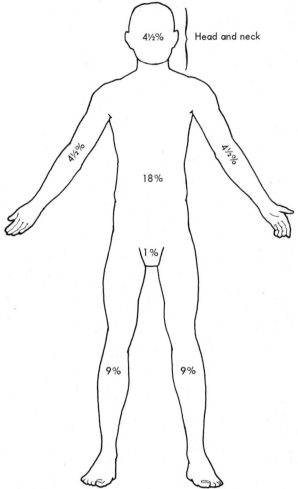

F IG. 9.   The rule of nines determines percentage of body involvement in the adult. The percentages shown above are for the anterior surfaces of the body. Those for the posterior surfaces are identical.

year until, at about age ten, it matches the 18 per cent of the adult. (See Table 10.)

Burns are considered "critical" if there is more than 30 per cent partial-thickness involvement or if there is more than 10 per cent full-thickness involvement.[7] If more than 20 per cent (10 per cent in children) of the body is involved, life is endangered. If more than 30 per cent is involved, the outcome is usually fatal.

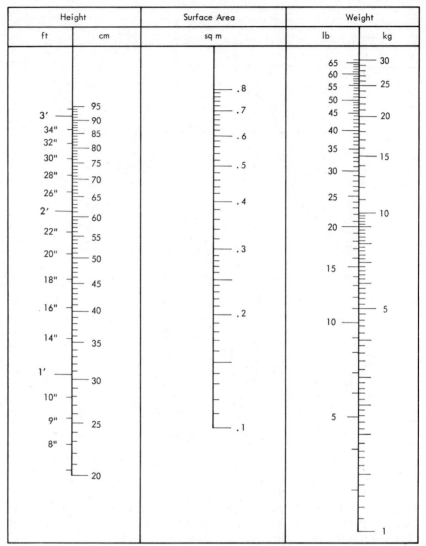

Height		Surface Area	Weight	
ft	cm	sq m	lb	kg

FIG. 10.   *A.* Nomogram for estimating surface area of infants and young children. To determine the surface area of the patient draw a straight line between the point representing his height on the left vertical scale to the point representing his weight on right vertical scale. The point at which this line intersects the middle vertical scale represents the patient's surface area in square meters. (Used by permission of Talbot, N. B.; Sobel, E. H.; McArthur, J. W.; and Crawford, J. D.: *Functional Endocrinology from Birth Through Adolescence,* Cambridge, Mass., The Commonwealth Fund, Harvard University Press, 1952.)

Height		Surface Area	Weight	
ft	cm	sq m	lb	kg

Height (ft): 7', 10", 8", 6", 4", 2", 6', 10", 8", 6", 4", 2", 5', 10", 8", 6", 4", 2", 4', 10", 8", 6", 4", 2", 3', 10", 8", 6"

Height (cm): 220, 215, 210, 205, 200, 195, 190, 185, 180, 175, 170, 165, 160, 155, 150, 145, 140, 135, 130, 125, 120, 115, 110, 105, 100, 95, 90, 85, 80, 75

Surface Area (sq m): 3.00, 2.90, 2.80, 2.70, 2.60, 2.50, 2.40, 2.30, 2.20, 2.10, 2.00, 1.95, 1.90, 1.85, 1.80, 1.75, 1.70, 1.65, 1.60, 1.55, 1.50, 1.45, 1.40, 1.35, 1.30, 1.25, 1.20, 1.15, 1.10, 1.05, 1.00, .95, .90, .85, .80, .75, .70, .65, .60, .55, .50

Weight (lb): 440, 420, 400, 380, 360, 340, 320, 300, 290, 280, 270, 260, 250, 240, 230, 220, 210, 200, 190, 180, 170, 160, 150, 140, 130, 120, 110, 100, 90, 80, 70, 60, 50, 40

Weight (kg): 200, 190, 180, 170, 160, 150, 140, 130, 120, 110, 100, 95, 90, 85, 80, 75, 70, 65, 60, 55, 50, 45, 40, 35, 30, 25, 20, 15

FIG. 10. *B.* Nomogram for estimating surface area of older children and adults. (From Talbot, N. B.; Sobel, E. H.; McArthur, J. W.; and Crawford, J. D.: *Functional Endocrinology from Birth Through Adolescence.* Cambridge, Mass., The Commonwealth Fund, Harvard University Press, 1952.)

The Inflammatory Response

The body's response to the trauma is inflammatory.[5] The capillaries dilate, and there is seepage of water, plasma, plasma proteins, and electrolytes (especially sodium) across the capillary membranes and into the burned area. It is hypothesized that damaged tissues contain large amount of macromolecules, with large surface areas on which water and ions are adsorbed,[8] further adding to the decrease in blood volume (hypovolemia) and the increase in interstitial fluid in the injured area. There is a concomitant decrease in water and electrolytes in the interstitial fluid in the uninvolved areas. The most rapid exudation occurs in the first six to eight hours; it may continue for 48 to 72 hours and may reach 1000 to 2000 ml a day.[5] Cells are damaged and potassium is released from them into the interstitial space. There is damage to the red blood cells, with clotting of cells in the wound area, and a generalized anemia. The

Table 10

CONTRIBUTION OF VARIOUS BODY AREAS TO TOTAL BODY SURFACES
AT DIFFERENT AGES BY PER CENT*

Area	Birth–1 yr	1–4	5–9	10–16	15	Adult
Head	19	17	13	11	9	7
Neck	2	2	2	2	2	2
Anterior trunk	13	13	13	13	13	13
Posterior trunk	13	13	13	13	13	13
Buttocks	5	5	5	5	5	5
Genitalia	1	1	1	1	1	1
Upper arms	8	8	8	8	8	8
Forearms	6	6	6	6	6	6
Hands	5	5	5	5	5	5
Thighs	11	13	16	17	18	19
Legs	10	10	11	12	13	14
Feet	7	7	7	7	7	7

*FROM Artz, C., and Reiss, E., *The Treatment of Burns*. W. B. Saunders, Philadelphia, 1957. Reprinted with permission. Adapted from Lund, C., and Browder, N., "The Estimation of Areas of Burns." *Surg Gynec Obstet*, **79**; 352–58, 1944.

large output of histamine from the damaged tissue can cause a shocklike reaction.

The Burn Phases

SHOCK: THE STAGE OF SODIUM LOSS

The shock phase lasts between 48 and 72 hours. This is an extremely dangerous period when fluids and electrolytes, particularly sodium, are being lost to the burn area and out of the body. Patients who feel well one minute suddenly become apathetic, nauseated, and weak. Urinary output often is negligible. The skin is cold and clammy, and there is a decrease in blood pressure with an increase in pulse rate. Patients may become disoriented. They may vomit blood.

The sequence of events is something like this:[9]

Injury from heat → increased capillary permeability → leakage of plasma proteins into interstitial space → decreased oncotic pressure of capillary → expansion of interstitial space and contraction of intravascular space → circulatory collapse.

Clinical shock is believed to be preventable if therapy can be instituted soon after injury.[9]

Much of the physiological derangement making up burn shock is related to the cellular effects of sodium deficit in unburned tissue.[8] Because of this, there seems to be a resurgence in the use of saline solution (i.e., Ringer's solution with lactate, pH adjusted to 8.2) in the treatment;[8] however, most authorities begin shock treatment with the use of colloid substances such as dextran, plasma, or whole blood in sufficient amounts to re-establish and maintain normal blood circulation. The most immediate need is to prevent circulatory collapse.

To help maintain kidney flow, Schumer[10] suggests intravenous infusion of 4 per cent urea in 5 per cent dextrose.

Patients are "monitored" by their urinary output, the goal being an output of 2 to 3 ml of urine per minute. If this monitoring is not possible (and it is not possible for children; it tends to overhydrate them), estimates must be made. For instance, fluids may be administered in quantity equal to 10 per cent of body weight if there are burns of 30 per cent or more, to balance loss of fluid in the wound edema. If the burn is extensive, blood and plasma may be used in equal amounts as the colloid replacement. In making calculations according to percentage of involvement, 50 per cent is used if the burn area totals 50 per cent or more.

The Brooke Army Medical Center Formula. The famous Brooke Army Medical Center formula is used frequently to calculate quantities of fluid and electrolytes for administration. It includes colloid, 0.5 ml per kilogram body weight times per cent of body burn; electrolytes (lactated Ringer's solution), 1.5 ml per kilogram body weight times per cent of body burn; water (glucose in water), 2000 ml; half of the total is administered in the first eight hours, and one fourth in the second and third eight-hour periods. Glucose is used as a protein sparer. In the second 24 hours, half the amount of colloid and electrolytes plus 2000 ml of water is used.[9] Potassium may be administered after the first 48 hours if there is adequate kidney function. The aim is to replace fluids and electrolytes lost from the vascular system in sufficient amounts to maintain perfusion of all tissues but not to administer so much fluid that there is added local edema.[11] Replacement is a delicate job. If overhydration is suspected, venous pressure is determined. No single formula meets the needs of all individuals. Formulas are only guides; the patient's condition and response to therapy are the main determining factors.

Therapy for Mrs. Brown during the shock phase included 500 ml dextran, 1500 ml lactated Ringer's solution, and 2000 ml glucose in water. She was not offered any tap water during the first burn day. Because she showed no evidence of peripheral vascular collapse, she was offered chilled hypotonic saline to sip.[12]

Vaporizational Heat Loss. One of the main problems is to reduce vaporizational heat losses from large burned areas. Some methods include continuous immersion in baths of controlled temperature; impregnating denuded areas with oleic acid to decrease water and heat loss; and continuous coverage of the wounds with thermo-pack dressings wet with chemical bacteriostatic agents such as 0.5 per cent aqueous solution of silver nitrate.[8]

It is possible that dressing large denuded areas with "normal" saline, which is not truly physiological, may cause sodium and water absorption in significant amounts.[13] Dressings using bacteriostatic agents must be so thick that they hold a large volume of solution and must be in contact with the wound at all points. These thick dressings should then be covered with dry cotton sheeting or a blanket to lessen evaporation and loss of heat through the dressing itself.[14]

THE POSTSHOCK PHASE: STAGE OF SODIUM AND WATER REABSORPTION AND DIURESIS

Treatment of the shock takes precedence over all other therapy. Once the shock is over, however, the patient must be observed closely for too rapid a diuresis with concomitant water-loss syndrome. Symptoms include thirst, dry mucous membranes, sudden loss of weight, apathy, or feeling of faintness. Both serum sodium and potassium must be maintained during this phase. As edema fluid is reabsorbed, pulmonary edema becomes a real possibility. Symptoms include feeling of chest constriction, a moist sound to the respirations, increased restlessness, and cyanosis of the nail beds.

The most serious problem to plague the burned patient for months after the shock phase is infection. The body's great barrier to infection, an intact skin, is broken. Bacteria gain entrance to the body easily and then find excellent growth media in the denuded areas. Bacteria survive and grow in sweat glands and hair follicles, even if the entire thickness of skin is nonviable. During the postshock period septicemia is the major cause of death.[15] If adequate prophylactic antibiotic therapy is given up to two months following the burn, beta-hemolytic streptococcus is rarely seen as the invading organism. Instead, *Staphylococcus aureus* and *Pseudomonas aeruginosa* are the culprits. Organisms beneath the burn eschar (dehydrated, dead skin) proliferate rapidly despite antibiotics.[11] Swab wipings of various parts of the body for culture help in the selection of appropriate antibiotics and determine their probable effectiveness. When the various catheters are removed, their tips are snipped off and cultured.[14]

Until the shock period is over, the patient is given nothing by mouth except a solution containing salt (4 gm per liter) and sodium bicarbonate (1.5 gm per liter) in iced water. If this is held, he is offered tap water and small amounts of fruit juice.[14]

Persistent negative nitrogen balance from loss of tissue with inadequate protein replacement results in increased susceptibility to infection and poor granulation-tissue formation.[9]

A high-protein, high-calorie diet beginning seven to ten days following the burn is suggested. This diet includes 2 to 3 gm protein per kilogram body weight, 50 to 70 calories per kilogram, 1000 mg vitamin C, 50 mg thiamine, 50 mg riboflavin, and 500 mg nicotinamide every day. Moyer and associates[8] suggest two multivitamin

capsules daily along with 4.8 gm calcium lactate and 10 to 30 ml
potassium gluconate containing 40 to 80 mEq potassium, three times
a day, by the third or fourth postburn day. An adequately treated
patient will gain weight the first 48 hours and then lose, so that he
will be below his preburn weight 7 to 12 days after the injury.[12]
Because of the negative nitrogen balance, some patients lose as much
as a pound a day for the first 30 days.[11]

Rapid removal of devitalized tissue, drainage, and early skin coverage, preferably with autografts but with homografts if the former
are not feasible, aid in the prevention of both infection and contraction. Research is being done to determine whether local application of
enzymes hastens the removal of burn eschar by penetrating and
destroying it.[10] Many authorities find that use of hydrotherapy
hastens the separation of the eschar.

There is some evidence that the toxic symptoms of burns are the
result of an antigen-antibody reaction and that, by administration of
burn donor sera, which can be stored at 4°C up to six months, the
toxic reaction is lessened.[10]

Implications for Nursing Practice

The care of the burned patient is complex and long-term. Because
each phase of the burn brings with it certain complications, the
nurse's astute observation is required, even when the patient begins
to look and feel better.

OBSERVATION

In the shock phase, there is a shift of extracellular fluids (primarily
sodium salts and sodium bicarbonate) from noninjured areas of the
body to injured areas, with resultant edema in injured areas and dehydration in the noninjured areas. The nurse must be alerted to signs
of dehydration and shock (restlessness, apprehension, thirst, feeling
cold, oliguria, poor tissue turgor, drop in blood pressure, increase in
pulse rate). It is important to keep a check on vital signs at least
every hour in the initial stage. Sometimes this presents a problem if
the most commonly used pressure points are involved. Blood pressure can be taken on the leg in the same way that it is taken on the
arm. The leg is stretched out (the patient can lie on his stomach if
possible), the cuff is applied on the thigh just above the knee, and

the stethoscope is placed over the popliteal space. The vital signs and the time should be recorded on a graphic sheet.

When the reabsorption phase begins, the nurse must be alerted to symptoms of pulmonary edema (moist sound to the breath, increased restlessness, cyanosis, feeling of chest constriction).

Because of the possibility of invasion by pathogenic organisms, she must watch for signs of infection and septicemia (temperature of 104 to 107°F rectally, rapid and regular pulse, hypotension, oliguria, paralytic ileus, disorientation, increased bleeding tendency, mild jaundice[7]). Medications, particularly antipyretics and antibiotics, should be given exactly on time and should be recorded immediately after administration so that the physician can compare vital signs with response to the medication.

The burned area is observed for amount and kind of drainage. Although there is no loss of fluid across the burn eschar, surprisingly large amounts of fluid collect underneath and surrounding the eschar. Until the crust is formed on about the third postburn day, all articles coming in contact with the burn should be sterile.

INTRAVENOUS THERAPY

Skilled planning of the intravenous regimen is a lifesaving measure for the severely burned patient. The physician orders the fluids and the sequence in which they are to be administered. It is the responsibility of the nurse to see that each bottle is numbered, labeled if medications or electrolytes are added, administered in the specific order requested by the physician, and recorded in the order administered. She regulates the intravenous drops per minute according to the span of time required for a quantity of fluid. For instance, if 2000 ml was to be given in 24 hours, it would run at about 21 drops per minute (see p. 150). The nurse checks the intravenous equipment frequently to make sure the tubing is not kinked, the drops per minute are regulated, and the fluid is not infiltrating. She reassures the patient and his family that this method of feeding is temporary, and she explains its purpose.

MEASUREMENT OF INTAKE AND OUTPUT

Particular attention is paid to all intake and output, and they are recorded carefully on a sheet provided by the hospital. Urinary output provides an indicator for the effectiveness of rate and quantity of intravenous administration. If the urinary output falls below 30 ml per hour (15 ml per hour in children), the intravenous drops per minute should be increased. If the output is above 50 ml per hour (25 ml per hour in children), the drops should be decreased. Volumes over 100 ml per hour indicate overloading[7] and should be reported to the physician immediately.

All output should be measured, or estimated, and recorded. This includes loss through burn drainage, perspiration, vomiting, sputum, bleeding, and stools. Urine not only is measured but is observed for appearance, gross blood, color, concentration, or dilution.

POSITIONING

In the early burn phase, elevation of involved areas aids in re-absorption of edema. The patient is turned and exercised to provide maximal exposure to the burned area. Cradles are used to keep the linen off the affected part and to provide some degree of warmth. The patient usually feels cold until the burn eschar forms. Heating lights are not suggested because they provide too optimum a temperature for microorganisms to grow. Splints made of various materials are used on the arms and legs to prevent flexion with contractures. Footboards are used to prevent shortening of the Achilles tendon. The trunk and hips are maintained in anatomical position, and the knees are extended. The elbow is kept extended with rolled towels, bath blankets, or small pillows. The wrist is extended and the fingers flexed with hand rolls. The shoulders are kept in anatomical position, except in burns of the axilla, where the shoulders should be abducted to 90 degrees.[7]

SPECIAL TREATMENTS

The nurse is responsible for carrying out many time-consuming treatments, vital to the patient's recovery. Often, wet dressings at a prescribed temperature are ordered to aid in débridement. The patient may be bathed in pHisoHex several times a day either in bed or in a tub. The temperature of the water in the tub must be checked frequently unless the tub has an automatic temperature control. Sterile linen in the room must be changed frequently.

NUTRITIONAL NEEDS

Adequate nutritional intake is vitally important for repair of damaged tissues. The patient often must be hand-fed, and the nurse's willing, patient attitude often is vital in ensuring adequate intake. If nutritional supplements are ordered periodically throughout the day, they should be offered at the right times. A high-protein milk drink would be too filling right after mealtime! Commercial supplements such as Nutrament (Edward Dalton Co.) and Sustagen (Mead Johnson Laboratories) contain several times as much protein as milk and are available in a variety of flavors.

Conclusion

Mrs. Brown was taken to the operating room soon after her admission for débridement of the burn areas. She was placed on intravenous therapy for five days. By the sixth postburn day she was allowed sips of salt solution and by the seventh postburn day sips of tap water and juice. By the eighth postburn day she was placed on a high-protein, high-caloric diet, with supplemental vitamins. Daily serum electrolyte studies and hematocrit determinations were done. Her intake and output were recorded. During the third postburn week autografts were taken from her thighs and were grafted to her chest and arm. She was immobilized for four days until the grafts "took" and then was encouraged to move. A regimen of physical therapy was planned and executed. Two months after her injury, Mrs. Brown returned home.

REFERENCES

1. COLLENTINE, G.: "How to Calculate Fluids for Burned Patients," *Amer J Nurs*, **62**:77, 1962.
2. RANDOLPH, J.; LEAPE, L.; and GROSS, R.: "The Early Surgical Treatment of Burns," *Surgery*, **56**:193, 1964.
3. BENNETT, H.: "Burns: First Aid and Emergency Care," *Amer J Nurs*, **62**:96, 1962.
4. SHULMAN, A.: "Ice Water as Primary Treatment of Burns," *JAMA*, **173**:1916, 1960.
5. GOLDBERGER, E.: *A Primer of Water, Electrolyte, and Acid-Base Syndromes.* Lea and Febiger, Philadelphia, 1959.
6. CONWAY, H.: "Management of Burns in Children," *Amer J Surg*, **107**:537, 1964.
7. BELAND, I.: *Clinical Nursing: Pathophysiological and Psychosocial Approaches.* The Macmillan Company, New York, 1965.

8. MOYER, C.; MARGRAF, H.; and MONAFO, W.: "Burn Shock and Extravascular Sodium Deficiency Treatment with Ringer's Solution with Lactate," *Arch Surg*, **90**:799, 1965.

9. ARTZ, C., and REISS, E.: *The Treatment of Burns*. W. B. Saunders, Philadelphia, 1957.

10. SCHUMER, W.: "Recent Advances in the Management of Burns," *Surg Clin N Amer*, **43**:229, 1963.

11. ARTZ, C.: "Recent Developments in Burns," *Amer J Surg*, **108**:649, 1964.

12. WEISBERG, H.: *Water, Electrolyte, and Acid Base Balance*. Williams and Wilkins, Baltimore, 1962.

13. MOSER, M.; ROBINSON, D.; and SCHLOERB, P.: "Transfers of Water and Electrolytes Across Granulation Tissue in Patients Following Burns," *Surg Gynec Obstet*, **118**:984, 1964.

14. MOYER, C.; BRENTANO, L.; GRAVENS, D.; MARGRAF, H.; and MONAFO, W.: "Treatment of Large Human Burns with 0.5% Silver Nitrate Solution," *Arch Surg*, **90**:812, 1965.

15. EDITORIAL: "Infection in Burns," *New Eng J Med*, **267**:363, 1962.

ADDITIONAL READINGS

ARTZ, C., and HOOPES, J.: "Current Knowledge of Fluid Balance in Burns," *Amer J Surg*, **103**:316, 1962.

BURKE, J.: "Boston Concept Uses Air and Plastic for Burn Isolation," *Mod Hosp*, **104**:80, 1965.

EDITORIAL: "How One Hospital Planned Its Burn Center," *Mod Hosp*, **104**:76, 1965.

EVANS, E.; PURNELL, O.; ROBINETT, P.; BATCHELOR, A.; and MARTIN, M.: "Fluid and Electrolyte Requirements in Severe Burns," *Ann Surg*, **135**:804, 1952.

GINSBERG, F.: "Management of Burned Patients Is Challenge to Aseptic Technique," *Mod Hosp*, **104**:114, 1965.

KEFALIDES, N.; ARANA, J.; BAZAN, A.; BUCANEGRA, M.; STASTNY, P.; VELARDE, N.; and ROSENTHAL, S.: "Role of Infection in Mortality from Severe Burns," *New Eng J Med*, **267**:317, 1962.

SECTION III

Replacement Therapy and Needs

CHAPTER 8

Replacement Therapy

ONCE the need for replacement therapy is determined, action must be taken promptly. Replacement must be instituted quickly, must be adequate to meet the needs of the patient, and must be sustained long enough for the body to re-establish water and electrolyte balance. Although sugar solutions, salt, and water were the main-stays of therapy not long ago, the goal today is a more sophisticated replacement of electrolytes as well as salt, water, and sugar.

The three main aims of water and electrolyte therapy are:

1. To replace previous losses.
2. To provide maintenance requirements.
3. To meet concurrent losses.

A detailed verbal history of recent intake and output is a vital adjunct in planning the therapy. Usually, sugar and salt solutions are used initially until kidney function is assured and laboratory tests indicate the more precise electrolyte needs.

The physician estimates the amount of fluid to administer either by age, by body weight, or by body surface area. The method of determining amount is controversial; the only established fact is that a relatively well-functioning body will adjust quantities admin-istered to its own needs, over a wide range of tolerances.[1] The follow-ing nomogram is used to determine body surface area. Derived from measurements of height and weight, it is expressed as square meters, M^2. A 50-kg (110-lb) woman, 5 ft, 2 in. tall, would have a surface area in square meters of 1.45. Abbott Laboratories chart the daily minimal, average, and maximal needs per square meter as shown in Table 11.

Table 11
NEEDS PER SQUARE METER BODY
SURFACE AREA IN A 24-HOUR PERIOD*

	Minimal	*Average*	*Maximal*
CHO		60–70 gm	
K	10 mEq	50–70 mEq	250 mEq
Na	10 mEq	50–70 mEq	250 mEq
H_2O	700 ml	1500 ml	2700 ml

*FROM *Fluids and Electrolytes*. Abbott Laboratories, North Chicago, 1960. Reprinted by permission.

Less chloride is required daily than sodium; for this reason, balanced solutions contain sodium salts of other acids as well as chloride.[2] Fluid is tolerated safely at $1\frac{1}{2}$ to 2 times the plasma volume, or roughly 5 per cent of body weight in kilograms, over a 24-hour period.[3] To keep a continuous check on the effectiveness of the treatment, weight is checked daily; intake and output are recorded; and laboratory studies, including determinations of red blood count, hemoglobin, hematocrit, and serum sodium, potassium, bicarbonate, and chloride, are done frequently.[4]

Methods of Replacement

Replacement methods fall under two broad classifications. The *enteral* route involves all feedings within the alimentary tract including the oral, nasogastric, and rectal routes. The *parenteral* route involves all feedings outside of the alimentary tract, including intradermal, subcutaneous, and intravenous feedings, intraosseous (into the red marrow of sternum or tibia), intra-arterial, and intra-peritoneal feedings.

THE ORAL ROUTE

The oral route is the method of choice. It is the normal route and is safest because it does not involve feedings directly into the blood stream with the ever-present possibility of overloading the circulatory system. There is also far less chance of an immunological reaction occurring.[5] But oral feedings must be planned and observed just as carefully as parenteral feedings!

TUBE FEEDINGS

If the patient is unable to take food or fluid by mouth because he is comatose, because of paralysis of the throat musculature, cancer of the mouth region, or gastrointestinal fistulas, or because he is senile and has lost the desire to eat, tube feedings may be indicated.[6] Gastric gavage involves the passage of a tube through the nose or mouth into the stomach. It is usually passed by a physician (some hospitals teach registered nurses the procedure) while the patient is lying on his side or while he is sitting with his head tilted slightly forward to help pass the tube along the floor of the nasal cavity.[6] There are several ways of checking whether the tube is in the stomach and not in the trachea. The tip of the tube may be placed in a glass of water; if it is in the trachea, bubbles appear as the patient exhales.[7] The physician may attach a syringe to the tube and withdraw gastric contents as an indicator. Polyvinyl is replacing rubber as the material of choice because it has been found to deteriorate less quickly, to maintain its softness and pliability for up to six to eight weeks within the stomach, and to be much easier for the patient to get down. Tubes that become rigid can cause trauma, with bleeding when they are removed.[6] When the patient's nutritional requirements are determined, special formulas are prepared and are dripped through the tube slowly at a rate of about 150 or 200 ml every three to four hours. No more than 500 ml is fed at one time.[7] The formula, made up of such items as eggs, milk, salt, vitamins, and Dextrimaltose, is diluted with water, warmed to 105°, and dripped through the tube slowly. It is usually preceded and followed by an ounce of warm water, also at 105°, to clear the tubing. Medications can be crushed and fed through the tube. The patient is fed while he is in an upright or semi-upright (45-degree angle) position to decrease the possibility of aspiration if the tube should become displaced. Mouth and nostril care with glycerin or half-strength peroxide should be given four to six times each day.

PROCTOCLYSIS

Proctoclysis, or feeding by rectum, is not used too frequently as it is difficult to ascertain exactly what has been absorbed. Water, sodium, and chloride are absorbed from the large intestine; food-stuffs are not.[5] Many hospitals have prepared proctoclysis trays (see a textbook on fundamentals of nursing for information concerning the Murphy or Harris drip). Usually, an enema is given one to two hours before the treatment. An 18-22 French catheter is inserted 4 to 5 in. into the colon, and the warmed solution is dripped through this tubing at a rate of 10 to 60 drops per minute,[7] or a total of 1000 to 2000 ml in 24 hours.

PARENTERAL ADMINISTRATION

The parenteral method, which is any method not involving the alimentary tract, is chosen because of its speed of action (intravenous), because a patient cannot take food or fluid by mouth, because the molecular weight of a particular drug is too large to have it absorbed through the gastrointestinal tract, or because the drug is destroyed by gastric juices.[8]

HYPODERMOCLYSIS

This is the subcutaneous route of administration, used when a vein cannot be entered or when infusion of fluid into the circulatory system is contraindicated.[5] It is often used in young children whose veins are small and difficult to enter and in older people whose veins are badly sclerosed.[9] Fluids are administered through one or two needles, directly below the layers of skin (not into the skin) but outside of the muscle tissue. A variety of sites can be used. These include the lateral chest, the abdomen midway between the navel and the anterior superior spine, the anterior and lateral aspects of the thighs, the loose tissue below each breast, the buttocks, and below the axillae. Clysis is fairly safe if the fluid administered resembles plasma in tonicity and contains some of the major ions of plasma.[10] Isotonic saline in water or dextrose, 2.5 per cent in half-strength saline, is a good example. Solutions lacking these ions cause extracellular water and electrolytes to diffuse into the clysis area, thereby decreasing plasma volume and possibly leading to shock.[4] Only isotonic or hypotonic solutions can be used. Frequently 150 units (15 to 1500 units) of an enzyme, hyaluronidase, is injected into the clysis tubing to increase the spread and thus enhance the absorbability of clysis solutions.[11] The enzyme must be used with caution as it can cause too rapid absorption of the infused fluid with overhydration. The enzyme is obtained from mammalian testes. It hydrolyzes the cement substance (hyaluronic acid) of connective tissue.[12]

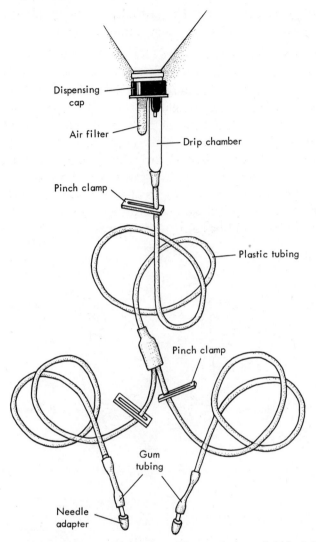

Dispensing cap

Air filter

Drip chamber

Pinch clamp

Plastic tubing

Pinch clamp

Gum tubing

Needle adapter

FIG. 11.   Hypodermoclysis. (Redrawn with permission of Abbott Laboratories.)

Dangers involved in administration by clysis include possible puncture of a large blood vessel, sloughing of tissue from lack of absorption of fluid, and infection with abscess formation. Clysis feeding is contraindicated for patients with subcutaneous edema.[13] Many hospitals use the commercially prepared clysis sets and attach needles $1\frac{1}{2}$ to 2 in. long, 19–22 gauge. The solution runs at a rate of

30 to 40 drops per minute. The procedure is too painful to have the solution run faster than the tissues can absorb it.[9]

INTRAVENOUS ADMINISTRATION (VENOCLYSIS)

The intravenous route is used when rapid absorption of a calculated quantity of fluid is required. It is lifesaving when blood volume must be replaced, as in circulatory shock. Fluids can be given for short or long periods of time, at rates of 30 to 60 drops per minute, or 60 to 120 drops per minute if the patient is in shock. All infusions are given slowly (not over 60 drops per minute) to patients with cardiovascular disease. The physician should determine the number of drops per minute, or the length of time a solution is to run. For instance, if 2000 ml of 5 per cent dextrose in water was to be given in 12 hours, it would be calculated this way:

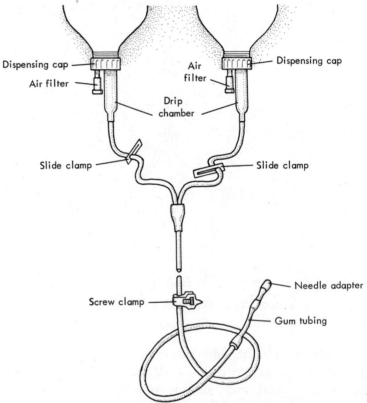

FIG. 12.   Y-type intravenous administration set. (Redrawn with permission of Abbott Laboratories.)

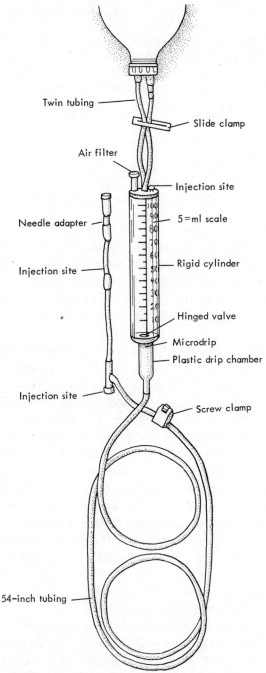

Twin tubing

Slide clamp

Air filter

Injection site

5 = ml scale

Needle adapter

Rigid cylinder

Injection site

Hinged valve

Microdrip

Plastic drip chamber

Injection site

Screw clamp

54-inch tubing

FIG. 13. Precision volume set with microdrip control. (Redrawn with permission of Abbott Laboratories.)

1. Read the directions of the commercial apparatus to see how many drops in each milliliter. There are usually 10 to 15 drops per milliliter in adult sets, 50 to 60 drops per milliliter in pediatric sets. There are 15 drops in each milliliter in the set being used for this calculation.
2. There are 15 drops in 1 ml; therefore, there are 30,000 drops in 2000 ml.
3. 30,000 drops: 720 minutes = x drops: 1 minute

   30,000: 720 = x: 1

   $720x = 30,000$

   $x = 30,000$ divided by 720

   $x = 42$
4. To have 2000 ml infused in 12 hours, regulate the drops at 42 per minute.

Several companies provide handy slide-rule-type calculators that determine drops per minute almost instantly. The companies will send them upon request. The rate of flow is influenced by the size of the needle, the height of the flask of solution, the viscosity of the fluid,[14] a shift in the patient's position, or anchoring tapes that are too tight.[15]

If a small, precise volume of fluid is to be administered, or if the rate of flow is to be slow, as for small children, special sets are available. When attached to the flask of solution, they control the volume by means of a specially calibrated cylinder or alter the number of drops that supply 1 ml of solution. The microdrip attachment supplies 1 ml in 60 drops. If the drops per minute were regulated at 60, the child would get 1 ml of solution; if the drops per minute were regulated at 60 in an adult set, he would get about 4 ml in a minute.

A scalp vein set, used for infusions in children and for infusions in small veins in adults, is pictured in Figure 14. It is a "thin-wall" needle, one in which the inside diameter is one size larger than the gauge.

Preparing the Infusion. If possible, the patient should be completely bathed, should have a clean hospital gown, and should have his treatments completed before the infusion is started. It is also a good idea, if feasible, to schedule the infusion so that it does not interfere with the patient's normal nighttime sleep.

Before setting up the equipment, read the manufacturer's directions carefully. Then attach the tubing to the bottle. If two bottles are set up at the same time, a Y-type administration set is used. If blood is to be administered, use only the blood administration set with its filter and bring along a small flask of normal saline to flush the tubing before and after the blood is administered. Bring the equipment into the patient's room, explain its use, and make sure the patient is identified accurately. The flask of solution is hung from an infusion standard about 12 in. above the level of the bed.[8] The newer beds store infusion standards with clamps behind the headboards and have openings in the head and foot of the bed for insertion of the standards.

Once the equipment is ready and the solution is allowed to run through the tubing to expel all air, the injection can be started. The nurse must be aware of the law of her particular state pertaining to who can administer intravenous infusions. She must also have adequate preparation in the principles of water and electrolyte therapy and supervision in the actual administration if she is to do the injection. Even if the state allows registered nurses to administer intravenous solutions, this does not exempt the nurse from liability if she attempts the procedure without adequate knowledge and preparation.[16] Many hospitals have a series of in-service classes to prepare nurses for this function. Schools are beginning to incorporate these principles and skills in their basic programs.

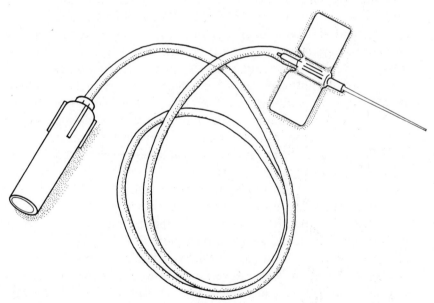

FIG. 14. Scalp vein infusion set. (Redrawn with permission of Abbott Laboratories.)

Choice of Site. Several superficial veins are suitable for intravenous infusions. The most frequently used veins are located at the inner aspect of the elbow in the antecubital space (basilic and cephalic veins) and on the dorsum of the hand (dorsal metacarpal veins.) They are easy to locate and enter and are most suitable for small injections that are not prolonged. The arm or hand is immobilized.

For long-term therapy, the accessory cephalic or median antebrachial veins, on the flat surface of the forearm, are used.[7] The saphenous vein at the ankle and the saphenous and femoral veins in the thigh, as well as the jugular vein in children, are also suitable. If a leg vein is selected, care is taken to avoid varicosities at or above the injection site. Varicose veins cause pooling or slowing down of infused fluid.[7]

The veins contain sensory nerves, and this accounts for the pain felt when they are pierced; however, with the exception of the discomfort of immobilization, there should be no pain once the initial injection is made.

Cut-Down. In some cases, especially in infants, when an assured route of fluid administration is required, a cut-down is done.[17] The saphenous vein at the ankle is often the site chosen. The skin is cleansed and anesthetized. A transverse incision is made through the skin over the vein, and the vein is brought into view. A small transverse incision is made into the vein, and it is cannulated with a catheter of polyethylene or other suitable material. The catheter should have the softness and flexibility of the vein so as not to produce mechanical trauma with limb motion and should be strong and durable because it often remains in the vein for long periods of time. Several sutures can be made to stabilize the vein, to anchor the catheter, and to close the skin wound.

The Injection. With the equipment set up and the flask of solution inverted on the intravenous standard, the operator is ready to inject the vein. The site is cleansed and the tourniquet is applied. A blood pressure cuff can be used, or a piece of rubber tubing tied in a slipknot or fastened with a hemostat is suitable. If the vein does not appear to dilate sufficiently, several measures can be taken. The arm can be allowed to hang dependent from the side of the bed; the vein can be gently slapped; or the arm can be wrapped in a warm, wet Turkish towel, covered with plastic, for 10 to 20 minutes.

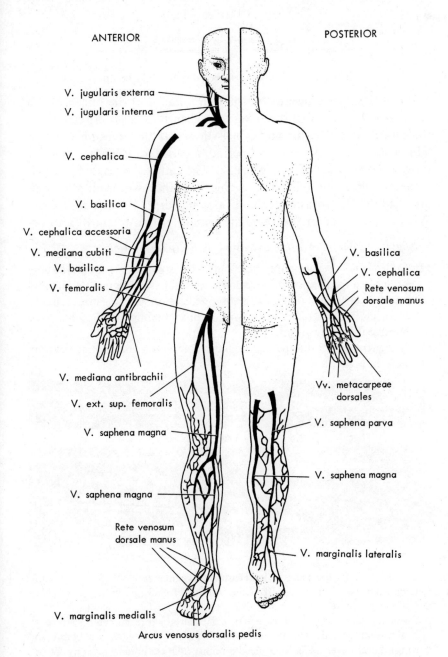

ANTERIOR

POSTERIOR

V. jugularis externa

V. jugularis interna

V. cephalica

V. basilica

V. cephalica accessoria

V. mediana cubiti

V. basilica

V. femoralis

V. basilica

V. cephalica

Rete venosum
dorsale manus

V. mediana antibrachii

V. ext. sup. femoralis

V. saphena magna

V. saphena magna

Rete venosum
dorsale manus

V. marginalis medialis

Vv. metacarpeae
dorsales

V. saphena parva

V. saphena magna

V. marginalis lateralis

Arcus venosus dorsalis pedis

FIG. 15.   The superficial veins used in blood transfusion or intravenous infusion. (Redrawn with permission of the Mayo Foundation.)

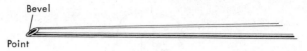

Bevel

Point

FIG. 16.   The bevel of the needle should be up.

When the needle inserted is small in relation to the lumen of the vein, it is inserted with the bevel up; when it is large in relation to the lumen of the vein, the bevel is down. If the solution is to be administered over a prolonged period, a catheter or cannula is often introduced in place of a rigid needle. The catheter is passed through a needle, into the vein. The needle is withdrawn from the vein, attached to the infusion tubing, and taped to the patient's arm. With the catheter in the vein, the patient is free to move around.

Suggested Steps in Administration of Solution by Vein.

1. Collect and prepare equipment outside the patient's room. Add any prescribed medication or vitamins and label flask. Equipment includes intravenous tray containing antiseptic, cotton balls, gauze squares, tape, etc.; flask of solution with proper tubing attached; arm or handboard for restraint.
2. Bring equipment into patient's room, identify him as for a medication, explain procedure.

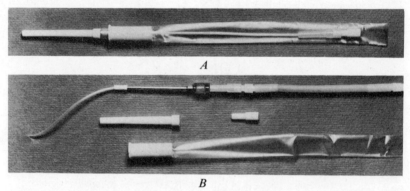

A

B

FIG. 17.   *A.* Bardic Deseret Intracath intravenous catheter placement unit. (Shown after aseptic removal from the Steril-Peel package, with needle guard and protective plastic catheter sheath.)
B. Intracath inserted. Sterile needle makes the venipuncture, catheter is advanced into the vein (plastic sheath maintains sterility, eliminates scrubbing and gloving), bevel cover slides over needle point; adapter attaches to any IV set. Assembly is taped to arm, the other three parts are discarded. (C. R. Bard, Inc. Murray Hill, New Jersey.)

3. Hang flask from IV standard. Attach needle to tubing; a 1 to $1\frac{1}{2}$ in., 18-19-20-gauge needle is usually selected. The more viscous solutions, like blood, require the larger bore. If a solution is to be given for a long period of time, a larger needle is chosen.
4. Allow solution to run through tubing and needle to expel the air.
5. Position the patient in flat or semiupright position.
6. Apply the tourniquet and select the vein. A vein that moves left or right at the thrust of the needle is not considered "stable."
7. Cleanse area with antiseptic and wipe off excess with dry gauze square to prevent sting of antiseptic introduced into the skin.[18]
8. Hold skin with one hand; introduce needle into the vein at a 30- to 45-degree angle. Most operators do not attempt to pierce the skin and vein in the same thrust. Abbott Laboratories suggests placing the tip of the needle slightly to one side of the vein and about 0.5 in. below the point where the needle will enter the vein itself; piercing the skin and underlying tissues to the depth of the vein, depressing the needle so that it is almost flush with the skin; moving it directly above and then into the vein.
9. After blood appears, advance the needle deep into the vein.
10. Release the tourniquet and begin the infusion.
11. Place a dry, sterile gauze square under and over the needle and tape the needle in place.
12. Restrain arm on armboard.

To Stop the Infusion.

1. Clamp infusion tubing; remove adhesive tapes by pulling toward needle.
2. Apply antiseptic-soaked gauze sponge or cotton ball on site of injection.
3. Gently draw needle out of the vein.
4. Continue to hold the sponge firmly in position, applying pressure, until all bleeding has stopped.[18]

Hazards of Intravenous Administration. Of the many complications arising from intravenous infusion, local reactions arising from trauma at the administration site are most frequently seen. If the wall of the vein is inadvertently pierced, discoloration and edema appear at the injection site, with infiltration of infused fluid into the tissue spaces and possible hematoma. The area around the injection site feels hard and is painful. If the condition is allowed to continue, there may be tissue necrosis. The vein is traumatized, too, if fluid is administered too rapidly in too small a vein.[7]

Thrombophlebitis occurs when the same vein is injected over and over again, when irritating or highly concentrated substances are injected,[8] or when a hooked needle is used. The vein hardens, and the patient experiences pain in the direction of the flow of blood.

When any local reaction occurs, the fluid should be stopped and a new injection site found.

Systemic Reactions. A pyrogenic reaction, in which the patient feels chills and has an elevated temperature, is most frequently seen.[7] It results from use of improperly sterilized equipment[8] or from pyrogen products of dead bacteria remaining in distilled water after being killed by sterilization. In an attempt to decrease the incidence of pyrogenic reactions, modern compression distillation equipment monitors the electrolyte count in distilled water and automatically diverts the flow of the distilled water if it contains over three parts per million of electrolytes.[19] Samples are studied to determine sterility, chemical content, and pyrogen content, and all bottles are checked visually for particles.[19]

Speed Shock. If fluids are administered too rapidly, the patient may experience pounding headache, chest constriction, chills, back pain, subcutaneous edema, rapid pulse, apprehension, dyspnea, and cardiac embarrassment. The fluid should be stopped immediately with the needle left in the vein, and the physician should be called. It is a good idea to anticipate his needs in the treatment of shock, with emergency drugs and equipment being made available.

Air Embolism. Though not seen too frequently, an embolism resulting from failure to clear apparatus of air before the administration of fluid may occur. The effects of the embolism will depend on which vessel is closed and on which tissues become deprived of their blood supply.[7] When arising from a venous thrombus, the embolus is likely to lodge in a vessel of the lung.[20]

Reactions occurring from the administration of blood are considered on pages 168-69.

Parenteral Solutions

WATER

An adult patient requires approximately 30 ml of water per kilogram of body weight (15 ml per pound). Thus a 60-kg adult requires 1800 ml daily. This requirement is increased when a person has fever or has excessive perspiration. Such persons require 2000 to 3000 ml daily in addition to the water lost via urine, which is 600 to 1500 ml. Water lost in vomitus, diarrhea, and suction needs to be replaced. Total body water per unit of weight is greater in infants than in adults, because the extracellular water volume is larger. Thus, infants and young children (up to 40 kg) require proportionately more water per kilogram of body weight than adults. Above 40 kg the water requirement is the same as for adults.

In the noningesting patient water is given by administering a 5 to 10 per cent glucose solution intravenously. Water alone cannot be infused as it will cause lysis of red blood cells owing to its hypotonicity. As soon as the glucose is metabolized or converted to glycogen, the water is readily available to the fluid compartment. Hypotonic saline solution may be used to replace water. This solution supplies proportionately more water than salt (0.45 gm of NaCl per liter); thus it is a means of administering water, while at the same time meeting salt requirements.

SOLUTIONS TO MEET CALORIC AND NUTRITIONAL REQUIREMENTS

Carbohydrate solutions are used to supply calories and to prevent ketosis. In the nonfebrile patient the average daily caloric need is about 1500 to 2500 calories. One hundred grams of glucose per day helps prevent the formation of ketone bodies. This amount can be supplied in 2 liters of 5 per cent glucose, or 1 liter of 10 per cent glucose.

Table 12
GLUCOSE SOLUTIONS

Solution	gm/L	cal/L
$2\frac{1}{2}\%$ glucose in water	25	85
5% glucose in water	150	170
10% glucose in water	100	340
20% glucose in water	200	680
$2\frac{1}{2}\%$ glucose in half hypotonic saline	25	85
5% glucose in 0.9% saline	50	170
10% glucose in 0.9% saline	100	340
10% glucose in Ringer's solution	100	680
50% glucose	500	1700

Invert sugar is a mixture of equal parts of fructose and glucose (levulose). Theoretically, the advantage of fructose over glucose is that it produces neither diuresis nor glycosuria and thus can be infused in higher concentrations.[11] However, there appears to be doubt among scientists as to whether fructose or invert sugar offers any real advantage over glucose.[21] Inasmuch as the provision of sufficient daily caloric requirements demands that a large volume (4 or more liters) of fluid be infused, a constant search is going on to find materials that will make abundant calories available that can be infused in a lesser volume of fluid. Alcohol and fat have been used intravenously to supply calories.

Table 13

INVERT SUGAR SOLUTIONS

Solution	Glucose, gm/L	Fructose, gm/L	cal/L
5% invert sugar	25	25	190
10% invert sugar	50	50	380
5% invert sugar in 0.9% saline	25	25	190
10% invert sugar in 0.9% saline	50	50	380

Alcohol is rapidly and completely metabolized, producing energy and sparing the body stores of fat, protein, and carbohydrate. A liter of 5 per cent alcohol in 5 per cent glucose yields 480 calories. In addition, alcohol solutions have a sedative and analgesic effect. Solutions containing alcohol are contraindicated in patients with kidney or liver disease.

Table 14

ALCOHOL SOLUTIONS

Solution	Alcohol ml/L	cal/L
5% alcohol in 5% glucose in water	50	480
10% alcohol in 10% glucose in water	100	960
5% alcohol in 5% glucose and amino acid solution	50	1000+

The intravenous administration of fat emulsions would provide a large part of the patient's caloric needs, as 1 gm of fat provides 9 calories. No thoroughly successful emulsified fat has as yet been made available. Cottonseed oil emulsion (Lipomul) has been used in patients with severe nutritional disorders, as in widespread malignancy.[6] Infusions of fat emulsions usually provoke unfavorable host responses. These untoward reactions may occur as early or late reactions. The early reaction is a severe shaking chill, accompanied by increased body temperatures—a side effect that defeats the advantage gained from the additional calories supplied, since an elevation of temperature sharply increases the caloric need owing to the accelerated metabolic activity. Another reaction that may occur early is the "colloidal" reaction. This is evidenced by lumbar pain, chest pain, dyspnea, cyanosis, urticaria, and hypotension. The late reaction, which appears in about three weeks, to the intravenous administration of emulsified fat consists of a rapidly developing anemia, rise in serum bilirubin, abnormal blood clotting, and hemorrhage from the gastrointestinal tract.[22] Patients receiving such infusions need frequent hematocrit determinations, blood coagulation tests, and serum bilirubin determinations. To date, a stable fat emulsion that can be tolerated when infused over any extended period has not been developed.[23] Emulsions of cottonseed oil and synthetic emulsions are currently under study. In fact, research is being carried on that will, hopefully, produce a single solution that will provide all the nutrients essential to life.

Proteins supply amino acids and nitrogen necessary for growth, tissue repair, and wound healing. If the patient is not able to take his protein requirement by mouth, the ideal way, and if he requires parenteral feeding over a period of time, it may be necessary to administer a protein hydrolysate intravenously. This should be administered with carbohydrate, which diminishes the utilization of amino acids as a source of energy and enhances the anabolic protein effects, such as tissue repair. Potassium must be a component of the preparation, as this ion is necessary for protein utilization for tissue synthesis. Parenteral administration of protein may evoke undesirable side effects, which include (1) a rise in body temperature, (2) nausea and vomiting, (3) severe headache, and (4) thrombophlebitis at the injection site. Protein solutions are contraindicated in patients with an allergic history or with renal impairment and advanced liver disease.

Table 15
AMINO ACID (AMIGEN) SOLUTIONS

Amigen Solution	Approximate Protein Equivalent (gm/L)[24]	Approximate Calories	Na, mEq	K, mEq	Ca, mEq	Mg, mEq	Cl, mEq	HPO₄ mEq	Lactate mEq
Amigen 5%	37–40	170	35	20	5	2	22	30	
Amigen 5% Glucose 5%	37–40	340	35	20	5	2	22	30	
Amigen 5% Levugen 10%	37–40	550	35	20	5	2	22	30	
Amigen 3⅓% Dextrose 3⅓% in ⅓ lactated Ringer's solution[5]	25–27	235	65	10	5	1	51	20	10
Amigen 5% Dextrose 5% Alcohol 5%	37–40	690	35	20	5	2	22	30	

Reprinted with permission from Baxter Laboratories, Inc.

Protein solutions administered intravenously are an enzymatic or acid digest of casein or beef and contain the essential amino acids.

SOLUTIONS PROVIDING ELECTROLYTES

Sodium Chloride Solutions. Sodium chloride solutions provide the chief cations and anions of the extracellular fluid. The important electrolytes of the intracellular fluid, such as potassium, magnesium, phosphate, and sulfate, are absent. Therefore, these solutions will not correct multielectrolyte deficits.

Isotonic Sodium Chloride. Isotonic saline solution (0.9 per cent sodium chloride) contains 0.9 gm of sodium chloride per liter. It is often referred to as "normal saline" or "physiological saline." This solution is neither normal in the chemical sense nor physiological, as it is hypertonic in relation to chloride as compared to extracellular water. Plasma contains 103 mEq of chloride per liter, while 0.9 per cent sodium chloride contains approximately 155 mEq per liter. It is, however, iso-osmotic and will not cause hemolysis of red blood cells.

Isotonic sodium chloride is used to supply salt, as in hyponatremia; to replenish chloride ion deficits, such as may occur in vomiting; to treat shock until other solutions are available (e.g., plasma or plasma expanders); and to treat oliguria.

Hypotonic Saline. One-half hypotonic saline (0.45 gm NaCl per liter) provides more water than salt for the body's use. This solution may be used to provide water while meeting the salt requirement.

Table 16

SODIUM CHLORIDE SOLUTIONS

Solution	gm/L NaCl	mEq/L Na$^+$	mEq/L Cl$^-$
0.9% sodium chloride ("normal" saline)	9	155	155
One-half (0.45%) hypotonic saline	4.5	77	77
Hypertonic saline 5%	50	850	850
Hypertonic saline 3%	30	650	650

Hypertonic Saline.   Hypertonic saline is available in strengths of 3 per cent and 5 per cent. Each liter of 5 per cent saline contains 50 gm of sodium chloride, and each liter of 3 per cent contains 30 gm of sodium chloride. It is indicated in severe salt-depletion states when rapid restoration is important without overloading of the plasma compartment with water. It is of value in treatment of states of water excess (water intoxication).

Sixth-Molar Sodium Lactate.   Sodium lactate (M/L) is used to treat moderately severe acidosis. The lactate ion is metabolized by the liver cells to bicarbonate, and sodium bicarbonate is formed. This solution is contraindicated in liver disease.

Sodium Bicarbonate Solution.   Sodium bicarbonate, 2 to 5 per cent in 5 per cent glucose, is used in severe metabolic acidosis.

Potassium.   Potassium may be administered either as potassium chloride or as potassium phosphate. The chloride salt of potassium is used more frequently. These salts are available in ampuls containing 20 or 40 mEq per ampul. The usual concentration employed is 40 mEq of potassium per liter. The required amount of potassium is added to 5 per cent glucose in isotonic saline. It is usually *not* added to electrolyte solutions, which already contain potassium.

Ammonium Chloride.   Ammonium chloride is an acidifying solution. The ammonium is converted to urea by the liver. The released chloride ions react with hydrogen ions, forming hydrochloric acid, which thus offsets a metabolic acidosis. Ammonium chloride is indicated where the metabolic acidosis results from vomiting with concomitant loss of hydrochloric acid. It is contraindicated in patients with impaired liver function, because the liver cannot convert the ammonium to urea, resulting in ammonia toxicity.

Special Solutions

RINGER'S SOLUTION

Ringer's solution is isotonic saline that has been modified by the addition of potassium and calcium in concentrations approximately equal to their concentrations in plasma. It may be used to treat hypohydration and loss of electrolytes and fluid as in vomiting, diarrhea, fistulous drainage, and gastric suctioning. It is usually considered to be prophylactic rather than therapeutic.

Lactated Ringer's Solution. Lactated Ringer's solution is similar to plasma in its electrolyte composition. In addition, it supplies lactate ions and is a useful solution to replace fluid losses. It is of particular value in the treatment of metabolic acidosis.

GASTRIC REPLACEMENT SOLUTION

This solution contains sodium and chloride in amounts equal to their concentrations in plasma. In addition, potassium ion is added in amounts similar to the concentration of this ion in intestinal secretions, which is approximately twice the concentration of this ion in plasma. Ammonium chloride is added to provide hydrogen ions and chloride ions, which replace the hydrochloric acid lost in gastric juice. The provision of hydrogen ion is made possible because the liver converts ammonium ions to hydrogen ions and urea.

Multielectrolyte Solutions

BUTLER'S SOLUTION

This solution contains:

Sodium	42 mEq/L
Potassium	30 mEq/L
Magnesium	5 mEq/L
Chloride	35 mEq/L
Bicarbonate	25 mEq/L
Phosphate	16 mEq/L

This is a mixed hypotonic electrolyte solution which provides water along with electrolytes.

DARROW'S SOLUTION

This solution contains:

Sodium	122 mEq/L
Potassium	35 mEq/L
Lactate	53 mEq/L
Chloride	104 mEq/L

This solution is intended primarily to replace fluid and potassium lost in infantile diarrhea and diabetic acidosis. Owing to the high concentration of potassium, this solution is contraindicated in improper kidney functioning.

TALBOT'S SOLUTION

This solution contains:

Sodium	40 mEq/L
Potassium	35 mEq/L
Lactate	20 mEq/L
Phosphate	15 mEq/L
Chloride	40 mEq/L

This solution is also a hypotonic multielectrolyte solution.

These three solutions are useful in treating mild to moderate multiple electrolyte deficits and in fluid replacement. They are contraindicated in severe electrolyte deficit; in severe burns, because of their high potassium content and their hypotonicity; in severe water loss, where water is required without electrolytes; in water excess; and in renal insufficiency.

Colloidal Solutions

Whole blood, plasma, packed red blood cells, packed plasma, concentrated salt-poor albumin, and colloidal plasma expanders such as dextran are available for increasing the circulating blood volume in blood loss and in shock.

Blood Groups

The bloods of different persons have different antigenic and immune properties, so that antibodies in the plasma of one blood react with antigens in the red blood cells of another. Furthermore, the antigens and the antibodies are almost never precisely the same in one person as in another. For this reason it is easy for blood from a donor to be mismatched with that of a recipient. When blood is mismatched, varying degrees of red cell agglutination and hemolysis may result. A person does not form immune bodies against the antigens in his own cells, but if cells from one person are transfused into another person, antibodies will be developed against all antigens not present in the recipient's own blood. Many of the antigens are common to many persons, and bloods are grouped or typed according to the major types of antigens present in the cells.

At least 30 commonly occurring antigens, each one of which can at times cause antigen-antibody reactions, have been found in human red blood cells. In addition to these, many hundreds of others of lower potency, or occurring in individual families, are known to exist. Among the 30 or more common antigens, some are highly antigenic and can cause transfusion reactions unless certain precautions are taken. The others are of importance for studying the inheritance of genes and thus are of value in forensic medicine.

Two particular groups of antigens are more likely than the others to cause reactions to transfused blood. These are the O–A–B system of antigens and the Rh–Hr system. Bloods are divided into different groups or types according to the antigens present in the red blood cells.

THE O, A, AND B ANTIGENS

Three different but related antigens—type O, type A, and type B— occur in the cells of different persons. Owing to inherited factors, a person may have one, or may have two simultaneously, but never all three. These three antigens are referred to as *group-specific substances*, because the different blood groups are determined by their presence or absence in the cells.

Type-O group-specific substance is very weakly antigenic; therefore, "anti-O" antibodies only very rarely develop in the plasma of any person. Type-A and type-B group-specific substances are strongly antigenic and cause severe agglutinative and hemolytic reactions. For this reason, A and B are called the agglutinogens.

Table 17

THE BLOOD GROUPS

Blood Groups	Agglutinogens	Agglutinins (alpha and beta)
O	—	α and β
A	A	β (beta)
B	B	α (alpha)
AB	A and B	—

Bloods are normally classified into four major groups (Table 17), depending on the presence of the two agglutinogens—A and B. When neither of these agglutinogens is present, the blood group is group O. When only type-A agglutinogen is present, the blood is group A. When only type-B agglutinogen is present, the blood is group B. When both A and B agglutinogens are present, the blood is group AB.

The Agglutination Process in Transfusion Reactions

When bloods are mismatched so that alpha or beta agglutinins are mixed with red blood cells containing A or B agglutinogens, agglutination occurs. In this process, the agglutinins attach themselves to the red blood cells, and because they are divalent, a single agglutinin can attach to two red blood cells, causing them to adhere to each other. This causes the cells to clump and thus plug small blood vessels. Subsequently, the reticuloendothelial system destroys these agglutinated cells, causing hemolysis with a resultant release of hemoglobin.

BLOOD TYPING

Prior to transfusing blood, it is necessary to determine the blood group of both donor and recipient, in order to ensure proper matching of blood. This is termed "blood typing." Two sera are required for typing, one containing alpha agglutinins and the second beta agglutinins.

Group-O red blood cells have no agglutinogens and, therefore, will not react with either the alpha or beta serum. Group-A blood contains A agglutinogens and therefore agglutinates with the alpha serum. Group-B blood contains B agglutinogens and therefore agglutinates with the beta serum. Group-AB blood has both A and B agglutinogens and therefore agglutinates with both sera.

CROSS MATCHING

An additional precaution to ensure compatibility of the bloods of recipient and donor is cross matching. This test consists of simply mixing the two bloods to determine whether or not agglutination occurs. If no agglutination of either the donor's or the recipient's cells occurs, it can be assumed that the two bloods are compatible.

THE RH AND HR FACTORS

In addition to type-O, -A, and -B antigens, red blood cells can contain other antigenic substances, including the "Rh factor." Blood containing this factor is termed "Rh positive," and blood not containing this factor is termed "Rh negative."

The Rh "Types" in Blood. The Rh system is very complex. Three major Rh factors have been isolated. These are the Rh_0, Rh′, and Rh″ factors. The red blood cells of 85 per cent of white persons contain Rh_0 factors, 70 per cent contain Rh″ factor, and 30 per cent contain Rh′ factor.

Rh negativity occurs principally in the white races; the different colored races tend to be almost entirely Rh positive. When the races are mixed, the incidence of Rh negativity increases. American Negroes, for example, are 95 per cent positive, because of the admixture of white blood.

The Rh_0 antigen is the only one of the Rh factors that is strongly antigenic; therefore, it is the one that is most often involved in transfusion reactions.

The Hr Factor. For each type of Rh factor there is a corresponding Hr factor—an Hr_0 factor, an Hr′ factor, and an Hr″ factor. These factors are almost never strongly antigenic and, therefore, rarely cause transfusion reactions.

OTHER BLOOD FACTORS

Many antigenic proteins besides the O, A, B, Rh, and Hr factors are present in the red blood cells of different people. They rarely cause transfusion reactions. Some of these blood factors are the M, N, S, s, P, Kell, Lewis, Duffy, Kidd, Diego, and Lutheran factors. The reader is directed to the references at the end of this chapter if further information is desired, especially the excellent review by Buchanan–Davidson.[25]

BLOOD TRANSFUSION

Whole-blood transfusions are required for hemorrhage, for shock due to hypovolemia, for coagulation deficiences, for exchange transfusions, and for extracorporeal circulation.

Packed red blood cells are used for anemic conditions. Transfusion with packed red blood cells prevents circulatory overloading. Lesser amounts of sodium and potassium and citrate ions are introduced into the recipient.

Hazards of Blood Transfusion. The main hazards of transfusions are the transmission of infectious diseases, hemolytic transfusion reactions, febrile reactions, allergic reactions, circulatory overloading, air embolism, and citrate toxicity. Untoward results from transfusions may also be due to errors in typing, cross matching, collection, or proper identification of donor and recipient.

Complications of Blood Transfusions. The immediate reactions to the transfusion of blood are febrile, allergic, circulatory, overloading, and hemolytic.

The febrile reaction consists of an increase in temperature with rigor. It generally occurs during the latter part of the transfusion or immediately thereafter. The allergic reaction is manifested by hives. Benadryl, Tacaryl, or some other antihistamine may be given concurrently with the transfusion in order to prevent this reaction.

Circulatory overloading is accompanied by a dry cough, engorged jugular veins, dyspnea, and cyanosis. It is uncommon but may occur if blood is given too rapidly to patients with some cardiac insufficiency. It is treated with tourniquets or venipuncture, digitalis, and oxygen.

The hemolytic reaction may be immediate or delayed. The immediate reaction appears early during the course of the transfusion and consists of lumbar pain, flushed face, hemoglobinemia, and hemoglobinuria. In the delayed reaction, the effects of hemolysis are revealed by jaundice. Toxic substances are released from the hemolyzed blood. These substances cause powerful renal vasoconstriction, which may lead to acute renal shutdown, renal failure, and death.

At any sign of a transfusion reaction, it is of vital importance to stop the transfusion immediately and notify the physician.

TRANSFUSION REACTIONS RESULTING FROM ANTICOAGULANTS

The usual anticoagulant for preventing clotting in banked blood is citrate. Citrate ions act as an anticoagulant by combining with the calcium ions of plasma so that these become un-ionized. In the absence of ionized calcium, coagulation cannot take place. Normal nerve, muscle, and heart function cannot occur in the absence of calcium ions. If blood containing large quantities of citrate is administered too rapidly, hypocalcemic tetany may occur. This reaction is most likely to occur when massive quantities of citrated blood are transfused. Hemorrhage, due to prolonged clotting time, is also a possible danger. In order to minimize the occurrence of these reactions, when massive transfusions are required, as in radical surgery for cancer, or cardiovascular surgery, heparinized blood or direct transfusion may be used.

TRANSFUSION REACTIONS DUE TO RH INCOMPATIBILITY

If the recipient has previously received a blood transfusion that contained a strongly antigenic Rh factor absent in his own blood, then he may have developed the appropriate anti-Rh antibodies against the Rh factor transfused. If a subsequent transfusion is given of the same type Rh blood, then an immediate transfusion reaction may occur. The characteristics of the reaction are almost identical to those that occur from mismatched blood groups.

If the recipient has never received a transfusion of Rh-positive blood, he will not have an immediate reaction. The antibodies require at least ten days to build up. If the Rh factor transfused is strongly antigenic, the titer of anti-Rh antibodies may be high. If such is the case, the slow agglutination and hemolysis of the infused cells result, causing jaundice, but no renal damage.

Plasma Transfusions

Plasma is sometimes equally as satisfactory as whole blood for transfusion. Properly matched whole blood is not always immediately available; moreover, valuable time may be wasted in typing, cross matching, and other serological studies. However, plasma can usually substitute very adequately for whole blood because it will increase the blood volume and restore normal hemodynamics. Plasma is used less in treatment at present because of the high incidence of homologous jaundice. If plasma that has been stored at room temperature for six months is available, it can be used without this risk. In the frozen state the virus is kept viable for indefinitely prolonged periods but soon loses much of its activity when kept at room temperatures.

Viral Hepatitis

Viral hepatitis is known to occur in two forms—that produced by the type-A virus (infectious) and that produced by the type-B virus (homologous serum jaundice). Both types may be spread from one person to another by transfusions of either whole blood or plasma. Type-A virus usually enters through the mouth but may be introduced parenterally. Type-B virus can only be introduced parenterally. The incidence of serum hepatitis is increased by the use of pooled plasma, which has been used in order to keep the titer of alpha and beta agglutinins low. The incidence of serum hepatitis has been reduced by pooling only a few units of plasma and storing at room temperature.

Dextran

Dextran is an artificial colloidal plasma expander. The hemodynamic benefits of dextran solution as a plasma expander are due to its colloid osmotic effect, by which the osmotic pressure of the plasma is increased, with resulting restoration of circulating blood volume. Dextran is available as a 6 per cent solution in isotonic saline. It is used to treat shock that results from hemorrhage, burns, trauma, severe dehydration, and surgical procedures. It is only administered intravenously. It can be given very rapidly at a rate of 1000 to 2000 ml per hour.

Patients may be hypersensitive to dextran. Urticaria, nausea, and vomiting, and even wheezing and shock, may develop. If this happens, the infusion should be stopped immediately. To prevent an allergic reaction, the infusion should be given slowly the first five minutes.[4]

LOW-MOLECULAR-WEIGHT DEXTRAN

Recently, dextran with a low molecular weight has been developed. When low-molecular-weight dextran is injected intravenously, it increases the colloid osmotic pressure of the blood. As a result, interstitial water is drawn into the blood, and the plasma volume increases. This result is transitory, lasting about 60 minutes, because low-molecular-weight dextran is rapidly excreted by the kidneys. It also decreases blood viscosity and sludging of blood and allows for greater blood flow through the capillaries. It is used when the hematocrit is high and the circulation is turning to sludge. Because of its ability to penetrate capillaries rapidly, it converts blood from a sol to a gel and reduces sludge formation resulting from decreased capillary blood flow.[26]

Low-molecular-weight dextran is still under investigation; it is being used only experimentally.

Nursing Implications of Parenteral Fluid Administration

PROTEIN SOLUTIONS

Protein solutions (Amigen) are started slowly and gradually increased. The beginning rate (adult) is 40 drops per minute, which is increased to not over 60 drops per minute. In children the rate is started at 10 drops and increased to 40 per minute. Nausea and vomiting may result from a too rapid rate of injection. Other medications are not to be injected into the administration set. If an allergic reaction occurs, the infusion is immediately stopped.

ALCOHOL SOLUTIONS

The patient who is receiving intravenous alcohol must be constantly attended and must be watched for stupor and signs of intoxication. The urine output must be accurately measured, and the nurse should be alert to any reduction in flow; if this continues, it should be reported. Intoxication can be avoided by regulating the rate of flow so that a 1-liter infusion is given in no less than four hours, a rate of flow of approximately 60 drops per minute. If sedation is also desired, the rate of flow may be 200 ml in 20 minutes (approximately 150 drops per minute); then one reduces the flow to the aforementioned rate. The site of injection is inspected freely in order to prevent leakage and infiltration into the surrounding tissues. Intravenous alcohol and sedatives, particularly barbiturates, are usually not administered together; therefore, nurses should not administer sedatives to these patients until they have carefully checked with the physician.

FAT SOLUTIONS

Fat solutions are still being used experimentally. The reason for continued and intensive research is that the solutions being tested can evoke a host of undesirable reactions. Since the solutions are still somewhat experimental, most nurses will not be participating in their use. Nurse practitioners who do work with them are, no doubt, members of a research team and are, therefore, more informed about their role. The nurse should be aware of the undesirable reactions, should stop the infusion at once if such reactions occur, or seem imminent, and should report the observation.

BLOOD TRANSFUSIONS

Blood is a tissue consisting of cells and extracellular substance, the plasma. When blood is transfused, the recipient is actually receiving the tissue of another person. Owing to the many factors that may be present in the donor's blood, there is always the possibility of an immune response by the recipient. Although the two bloods have been typed and cross-matched, the potentiality exists that there may be some factor in the donor's blood that the laboratory tests have failed to reveal. If such a factor is present, it may evoke an immune response, especially if the unrevealed factor is strongly antigenic. Therefore, all patients receiving blood, and especially those who require several transfusions, must be carefully watched for signs of a transfusion reaction. If any such signs appear, the transfusion must be stopped at once.

How to Administer Blood

When the blood comes from the blood bank, it is in a plastic or glass container, labeled clearly as to type, Rh factor, date drawn, use of anticoagulant-preservative (acid citrate–dextrose), and expiration date. It has been collected by the indirect method (donor to flask; flask to recipient) and has been refrigerated up to 21 days at 4 to 10°C (39 to 50°F). It is dark red and should contain no air bubbles. It is ready for use.

Whole blood or its fractions are administered by gravity drainage directly into the circulatory system. If a plastic container is used, the bag compresses as it empties. It is never air-vented. If a glass bottle is used, it is vented with an air-vent needle once the administration has started. This clears any blood present in the air tube. Because red cells tend to settle to the bottom and plasma rises to the top, the blood is thoroughly mixed prior to the infusion and then periodically agitated during the infusion.

The patient is identified carefully to make sure the blood is actually meant for him. His blood type, found on the chart, is compared with the type found on the label of the bottle of blood.

The blood is administered from a primary bottle with a single length of tubing, or from a secondary bottle using a Y-type administration setup. It can be immediately preceded by a solution that does not contain calcium. A calcium-containing solution will cause hemolysis, clumping of cells, or untoward reaction when mixed with blood. If such a solution must precede the administration of blood, the tubing must be thoroughly flushed with normal saline before the blood is started. Isotonic sodium chloride or dextrose, 5 per cent in quarter- or half-strength saline (not plain 5 per cent dextrose), is compatible with blood. A small flask of isotonic saline is often used routinely to flush the tubing and to make sure that the needle is well situated in the vein before the blood is started.

If a Y-type setup is used, the solution from only one of the bottles can run into the vein at one time. Tubing to the other bottle must be tightly clamped. To decrease the possibility of an air embolism, neither bottle is allowed to empty fully.

Only a blood administration tubing set with its filter can be used for the administration of blood.

The drip chamber is filled just enough to cover the filter before infusion is started. If the filter becomes clogged, it is cleared by squeezing the flexible drip chamber above the filter after the clamp has been closed. If the drip chamber assumes an "hourglass" shape, the airway is plugged and the air-vent needle must be replaced.

If the blood is to be administered rapidly, a setup containing a bulb pump can be used. When the pump is squeezed, blood enters the vein rapidly. When it is not squeezed, the original rate is resumed.

Because blood is made up of large molecules and is a viscous solution, a large enough needle must be selected for use. A No. 18

regular needle or No. 19 thin-wall needle is suitable. The first 50 ml is administered slowly in the first half hour. The nurse stays with the patient continuously the first 15 to 30 minutes to observe for signs of incompatibility. The rate is then regulated by the physician's orders, usually between 30 and 60 drops per minute.

REFERENCES

1. WEISBERG, H.: *Water, Electrolyte and Acid-Base Balance.* Williams and Wilkins Company, Baltimore, 1962.
2. ABBOTT LABORATORIES: *Fluids and Electrolytes.* North Chicago, Ill., 1960.
3. LOWE, C.: "Principles of Parenteral Fluid Therapy," *Amer J Nurs,* **53**:963, 1953.
4. GOLDBERGER, E.: *A Primer of Water, Electrolyte and Acid Base Syndromes.* Lea and Febiger, Philadelphia, 1959.
5. ELKINTON, J., and DONOWSKI, T.: *The Body Fluids: Basic Physiology and Practical Therapeutics.* Williams and Wilkins, Baltimore, 1955.
6. DAVENPORT, R.: "Tube Feeding for Long Term Patients," *Amer J Nurs,* **64**:121, 1964.
7. SUTTON, A.: *Bedside Nursing Techniques in Medicine and Surgery.* W. B. Saunders, Philadelphia, 1964.
8. ABBOTT LABORATORIES: *Parenteral Administration.* North Chicago, Ill., 1959.
9. MONTAG, M., and SWENSON, R.: *Fundamentals in Nursing Care.* W. B. Saunders, Philadelphia, 1961.
10. WOLF, E.: "The Nurse and Fluid Therapy," *Amer J Nurs,* **54**:831, 1954.
11. BECKMAN, H.: *Drugs, Their Nature, Action, and Use.* W. B. Saunders, Philadelphia, 1958.
12. MUSSER, R., and SHUBKAGEL, B. L.: *Pharmacology and Therapeutics,* 3rd ed. The Macmillan Company, New York, 1965.
13. PRICE, A.: *The Art, Science, and Spirit of Nursing.* W. B. Saunders, Philadelphia, 1965.
14. McLAIN, M., and GRAGG, S.: *Scientific Principles in Nursing.* C. V. Mosby, St. Louis, 1962.
15. SHANCK, A.: "The Nurse in an Intravenous Therapy Program," *Amer J Nurs,* **57**:1012, 1957.
16. PLANT, M.; IVERSON, L.; BARBEE, G.; SCOTT, W.; and SMITH, D.: "Nursing Practice and Intravenous Therapy," *Amer J Nurs,* **56**:572, 1956.
17. NELSON, W.: *Textbook of Pediatrics.* W. B. Saunders, Philadelphia, 1959.
18. JOHNSON, L.; GILLIS, S.; and LYNN, H.: "Unusual Complication of Intravenous Fluid Therapy," *Surgery,* **53**:809, 1963.
19. SHERMAN LABORATORIES: *Intravenous Solutions, Disposable Administration-Equipment, Blood Donor and Administration Units.* Detroit, 1964.
20. BEST, C., and TAYLOR, N.: *The Physiological Basis of Medical Practice,* 6th ed. Williams and Wilkins, Baltimore, 1955.

21. GRACE, W.: *Practical Clinical Management of Electrolyte Disorders.* Appleton-Century-Crofts, New York, 1960.
22. LEHR, H.; RHOADS, J.; ROSENTHAL, D.; and BLAKEMORE, W.: "The Use of Intravenous Fat Emulsions in Surgical Patients," *JAMA,* **181**:745, 1962.
23. COHN, I.; SINGLETON, S.; HARTWIG, Q.; and ATIK, M.: "New Intravenous Fat Emulsion," *JAMA,* **183**:755, 1963.
24. DONALDSON, R., and PALETTA, F.: "An Improved Method of Direct Cannulation of the Carotid Artery for Infusion," *Amer J Surg,* **106**:712, 1963.
25. BUCHANAN-DAVIDSON, D.: "A Drop of Blood," *Amer J Nurs,* **65**:103, 1965.
26. GELIN, L.; SALVELL, L.; and ZEDERFELDT, B.: "The Plasma Volume Expanding Effect of Low Viscous Dextran and Macrodex," *Acta Chir Scandinav,* **122**:309, 1961.

ADDITIONAL READINGS

ABBOTT LABORATORIES: *The Use of Blood.* North Chicago, Ill., 1961.
ALLEN, J.; EVERSON, D.; BARON, E.; and SYKES, C.: "Pooled Plasma with Little or No Risk of Homologous Serum Jaundice," *JAMA,* **154**:103, 1954.
AMERICAN HOSPITAL SUPPLY CORPORATION: *Blood Bank Procedures.* Evanston, Ill., 1952.
C. R. BARD, Inc.: *Products for Intravenous Infusion.* Murray Hill, N.J., 1965.
DARROW, D.: "The Physiologic Basis for Estimating Requirements for Parenteral Fluids," *Pediat Clin N Amer,* **6**:282, 1959.
EDITORIAL: "Pooled Plasma and Jaundice," *JAMA,* **154**:146, 1954.
GRONWELL, A.: *Dextran and Its Use in Colloidal Infusion Solutions.* Academic Press, New York, 1957.
HAYNES, B.: "Dextran Therapy in Severe Burns," *Amer J Surg,* **99**:684, 1960.
KNISELY, M.; ELIOT, T.; and BLUEC, E.: "Sludged Blood in Traumatic Shock," *Arch Surg,* **51**:220, 1945.
LONG, D.; SANCHEZ, I.; VARCO, R.; and LILLIHEI, C.: "The Use of Low Molecular Weight Dextran and Serum Albumin in Extracorporeal Circulation," *Surgery,* **50**:12, 1961.
McGAW LABORATORIES: *A Guide to Parenteral Fluid Therapy.* Glendale, Calif., 1963.
NEALON, T.; CHENG, N.; and GIBBON, J.: "Prevention of Citrate Intoxication During Exchange Transfusions," *JAMA,* **183**:459, 1963.
RACE, R., and SANGER, R.: *Blood Groups in Man.* Charles C Thomas, Springfield, Ill., 1962.
SHILS, M.: "Intravenous Fat Administration," *New York J Med,* **60**:2200, 1960.
SMITH, D.; KLOPP, C.; and ALFORD, C.: "Present Status of Isolation Perfusion and Intraarterial Infusion Technics," *Postgrad Med,* **32**:135, 1962.
SOULIER, J.: "Transfusion Reaction," *Blood,* **7**:664, 1952.
STEWART, R., and SANISLOW, C.: "Silastic Intravenous Catheter," *New Eng J Med,* **265**:1283, 1961.

CHAPTER 9

Water and Electrolyte Needs of the
Young and Old

Immortality requires a continuously ideal environment.   STEIGLITZ

THE two extremes of life present problems relative to the age of the patient that influence water and electrolyte metabolism. The very young have wide fluctuations in several physiological constants, while the aged have a much narrower margin of safety owing to decreasing ability to withstand the stress of injury and illness. It has been said that homeostatic function throughout the life-span can be compared to a funnel, with the wide top of the cone representing the very young and gradually narrowing through the years to the pipelike end, which represents the elderly.

The Young Child

Total body water per unit of weight is greater during infancy than in later life. The relatively large body-water volume of infants is due to a large extracellular volume. From birth until about two years of age there is a gradual decrease of extracellular and total body water. Although total body water is greater in infants than in older children and adults, infants do not have a surplus of water. The intake and excretion of water per kilogram of body weight are greater in the infant, the daily turnover amounting to half his extracellular fluid volume. The reasons for this are: (1) The basal heat production per kilogram of body weight is twice as high in infants as in adults. Because of this metabolic factor, and because infants have a greater total body surface in proportion to their size, they lose twice as much water per kilogram as do adults. (2) Because of this greater metabolic

176

rate, there is an increase in the metabolic end products, with a relatively larger amount of water being required to excrete these in the urine. Because of this high rate of turnover of water, any fluid loss or lack of intake depletes the infant's extracellular water volume rapidly.

The most important difference between young children and adults with a disorder in water-and-electrolyte balance is in body size and fluid composition and the concomitant speed with which imbalances occur. An infant in optimum health can be severely dehydrated after a day of vomiting. A child with infantile diarrhea and vomiting together will go into hypovolemic shock with alarming speed.

Little is known about exact fluid requirements for the premature and term infant, though approximation of various needs has been made. On the basis of the child's weight, body surface area, recent history of weight loss, and amount of fluids lost and gained, the physician orders the fluid to be administered. Because it is so easy to overhydrate the infant, or to introduce electrolytes in excess of need, it is better to give too little than too much solution in meeting maintenance requirements.[1] If possible, the total daily volume of intravenous solution should be administered over a 24-hour period; however, if this is impractical, the total requirements can be given in three or four divided doses spaced at regular intervals throughout the allotted time span. The same kinds of replacement solutions are used for the child and for the adult; however, the young child is frequently given half-strength solutions rather than full-strength solutions, and the quantities are, of course, smaller. The reader is requested to see Chapter 8 for description of commercial apparatus available for administration of fluids to children.

The importance of astute, knowledgeable observation by the nurse cannot be overemphasized. Because she can make comparison observations over an extended period of time, she can frequently distinguish minor changes in behavior, in vital signs, and in general appearance that might forewarn against dire imbalance. Her actions can be lifesaving!

The Infant with Salicylate Poisoning

Mr. and Mrs. Jones are a well-educated couple who take the utmost care to prevent accidental poisoning of their children. Their household detergents and powders are stored in high cabinets rather than under the sink; their drugs are kept in a locked medicine chest. One evening, two-year-old Janie had a cold, and Mr. and Mrs. Jones had theater tickets. They were late. Mrs. Jones took out the orange-flavored aspirin and left it on the sink. When the teen-age baby sitter arrived, Mrs. Jones told her to give the child one baby aspirin before bedtime. Then, to avoid entering the theater after curtain time, the well-bedecked couple left the house without further instructions to the baby sitter.

What happened in the next six hours is obscure; however, when the couple returned, the aspirin bottle was not on the sink, and they forgot about it entirely.

During the following two days the child had periods of vomiting and diarrhea. She was admitted to the hospital, at which time her stools were watery, and her urine was scanty and very concentrated. The physical examination revealed a temperature of 102.6°F, a pulse rate of 150, and a respiratory rate of 52 per minute. The admitting diagnosis was gastroenteritis of unknown origin. Initial orders were:

Vital signs q. 2 h.
N.P.O.
C.B.C.
Hematocrit
Serum chlorides, potassium, sodium, urea nitrogen
Urinalysis
5% dextrose in half-strength saline, 1500 ml, at 60 microdrops per minute

At 7 P.M. on the evening of admission the nurse noted that the child was becoming increasingly restless, and irritable and was in severe distress, with respirations of 84 per minute. The house physician was notified of the change in condition. After examining the child, he wrote a note on the chart that he suspected either metabolic acidosis or respiratory alkalosis, from salicylate poisoning. Salicylate intoxication often causes a mixed condition in which there is metabolic acidosis followed by respiratory alkalosis. Initially, the salicylic acid anions cause a decrease in extracellular bicarbonate, hydrogen ion concentration rises (pH falls), and metabolic acidosis occurs. Then, the low pH, if not corrected, stimulates the respiratory center so greatly that there is a decrease in extracellular carbonic acid with resultant alkalosis. The following orders were written:

Blood pH, carbon dioxide combining power, and blood salicylate level
 stat
Urine pH stat

The blood pH was 7.270, urine pH 5, carbon dioxide combining
power 28 volumes per cent, and salicylate level 66 mg per cent. These
findings are indicative of metabolic acidosis caused by salicylate
ingestion.

When the mother was questioned, she remembered the lost bottle
of baby aspirin but could give no estimation of the number of aspirin
the child had taken.

At this point, the major goal in treatment focused on reversing the
metabolic acidosis and providing sufficient parenteral fluids to
prevent underhydration. The orders were:

Bicarbonate, 22 mEq in 250 ml of $\frac{1}{3}$ saline, with 5% dextrose—60 microdrops per minute. This order to be repeated once.

At midnight the temperature was 103.2°F, pulse 130, and respirations
60 per minute. The child was in less acute distress, and urinary output
was increasing. She was less irritable.

At 8 A.M. of the day following admission the temperature was
100.6°F, pulse 130, and respiratory rate 32 per minute. The child was
crying almost continuously. Oral fluids were ordered and retained.
Diarrhea had ceased, and urinary output was satisfactory. The
salicylate level was 46 mg per cent, blood pH was 7.445, and the
carbon dioxide combining power was 31 volumes per cent. Ionosal
MB (Abbott Laboratories), containing dextrose, magnesium chloride
anhydrous, potassium chloride, monopotassium phosphate anhydrous, monosodium phosphate anhydrous, and sodium lactate
anhydrous, 1500 ml at 60 microdrops per minute, was ordered, and
oral fluids were continued. In the afternoon the child was put on a
soft diet, which she retained.

On the second day following admission vital signs were normal,
the child was retaining the soft diet and voiding, and the blood
salicylate level was 3.9 mg per cent. Intravenous fluids were discontinued, and oral fluids were encouraged. Two days later the infant
was discharged.

This was a fortunate situation in which water and electrolyte
therapy prevented irreversible central nervous system changes, coma,

Table 18
CONCENTRATIONS OF ANIONS AND CATIONS
OF NORMAL SERUM OR PLASMA*

Ion	Range, mg/100 ml	Range, mEq/L
Chloride		
Premature infants	353–440	99–124
Full-term infants	355–386	100–109
As sodium chloride	560–630	98–108
CO_2 combining capacity 55–70 vol %		22–30
CO_2 content		
Premature infants	24.0–60.8	10.9–29.1
Full-term infants	24.7–56.0	11.2–24.1
4 to 24 hours old	31.2–54.8	14.2–24.9
1 to 5 days old	38.0–66.3	17.2–30.1
Protein	gm/100 ml	
Premature infants	4.1–6.5	10.0–15.7
Full-term infants	5.7–6.7	13.7–16.3
Phosphate (as phosphorus)	mg/100 ml	
Children	4.0–6.0	2.3–3.6
Sulfate (as sulfur)	1.6–2.4	1.0–1.5
Undetermined anions		4–6
Total anions		145–157
Sodium		
Full-term infants	295–350	128–152
Potassium		
Full-term infants	14–22	3.5–5.6
Calcium		
1 to 7 days old	7.5–13.9	3.5–6.8
1 to 24 months old	9.4–11.5	4.7–5.8
Magnesium		
Premature infants		152–171
Full-term infants		148–159
4 to 24 hours old		147–160
Hydrogen (pH units)		
Premature infants		7.18–7.48
Full-term infants		7.20–7.48
4 to 24 hours old		7.33–7.50
1 to 5 days old		7.25–7.59

*FROM Armstrong, I. L., and Browder, J. J., *The Nursing Care of Children.* F. A. Davis, Philadelphia, 1964. Reprinted with permission.

and death. If the child had been brought to the hospital immediately after she ingested the aspirin, prompt gastric lavage might have eliminated the need to administer parenteral infusions. If the intake of salicylate had been very severe, exchange transfusions or peritoneal dialysis might have been needed. Needless to say, this intelligent couple neglected a vital area of baby-sitter education. Though they were knowledgeable themselves, they left their child in the care of someone who was not, and in their haste to leave the house, they were unsafe in their practices. Their child suffered the consequences.

The Geriatric Patient

The aging process is characterized by changes in structure, gradual decrease in body functions, and decrease in the ability to recuperate from injury and stress. The primary problem of aging is the maintenance of homeostatic mechanisms, specifically the excretion of end products of metabolism. Diminished pulmonary, cardiac, and kidney function leads to the accumulation of metabolic waste products. These factors render the aged patient vulnerable to water-and-electrolyte imbalances, accompanied by the inability to regulate these imbalances.

THE RESPIRATORY SYSTEM

In the aged person the chest walls are rigid, and there are reduction of maximal breathing capacity and loss of elasticity of parenchymal lung tissue. There is poor diffusion of respiratory gases owing to defective alveolar ventilation. Accumulation of bronchial secretions tends to occur, which further reduces ventilation and leads to obstructive emphysema. These deficiencies lead to decreased carbon dioxide elimination and place the older patient in a state of impending respiratory acidosis.

Breathing exercises and positioning that allows for maximal chest expansion and coughing are important measures that help the patient to improve his breathing capacity and to increase the elimination of carbon dioxide. The patient often breathes more readily in the sitting position. Adequate support must be supplied, and the head should be in such a position that the chin does not rest on the chest. Allowing the patient to sit forward, resting on an over-bed table, will allow for maximal chest expansion. In positioning a patient in a chair, good body alignment should be maintained and the arms supported. If the patient is permitted to slump in a chair, breathing capacity will be reduced. Breathing exercises include not only deep inspiration but also prolonged expiration in order to increase carbon dioxide removal. Exercises for the older patient should be scheduled and supervised so that they are not neglected and forgotten.

THE KIDNEYS

In aging, there is a gradual decrease in renal function. This is due to a persistent renal vasoconstriction, reduced glomerular filtration rate, and decrease in the amount of functioning tissue. This reduction of function gives rise to a loss of ability to excrete or to retain water and solutes as the need arises. This is especially critical in relation to hydrogen ion regulation. In the older person the blood becomes more acidic, and as anemia is quite common in the aged, there is loss of the important buffer hemoglobin. These factors increase the plasma concentration of hydrogen ion. Coupled with this is the decreased ability of the kidney to regulate hydrogen ion excretion. Thus the elderly patient may quickly develop a metabolic acidosis.

DEHYDRATION

In younger persons, the thirst mechanism serves as an indicator of the need for water. In the aged, this mechanism may be decreased or absent. There may be forgetfulness or mental confusion, or the patient may be too ill or too weak to ask for water or to lift the bedside carafe. This leads to grossly insufficient intake. The renal tubular cells are less able to concentrate urine, and there is a diminished response by these cells to antidiuretic hormone with the result that a dilute urine is formed and excreted. These two factors, insufficient intake of water and increased output, render the aged patient highly susceptible to dehydration. Adequate amounts of water should be supplied and the patient frequently reminded or assisted to drink water. If the dehydration is severe, fluids are given intravenously to replace the deficit.

SURGERY IN THE AGED PATIENT

Ideally, surgery in the aged requires as much attention to preoperative preparation as to postoperative care. Unfortunately, much surgery in this age group is of an emergency nature. If there is time to adequately prepare the patient, the nurse should have knowledge as to the type of surgery to be performed and should plan with the surgeon regarding the appropriate preoperative regime. The aged are handicapped by retarded healing and regenerative capacities, reduced margins of safety in the various organ systems, and numerous nutritional deficiencies.

Weighing the patient preoperatively is important. In the older patient weight loss after surgery may be marked. Knowing the preoperative weight is essential in the estimation of the degree of postoperative weight loss. The aged are particularly vulnerable to water intoxication. This is most likely to occur the first two days after surgery, when oliguria is present and parenteral fluids are being administered. This condition is accompanied by weight gain, which cannot be estimated unless the preoperative weight is known. Weights taken on successive days at the same time and after the patient has voided are more accurate and provide the physician with more information than a single weight.

In order to know whether the preoperative volume of urine is adequate, the output should be measured. Postoperative oliguria is more marked in the old than in the young. Oliguria during the first 48 hours postoperatively is a good sign, especially when it is known that the preoperative output was adequate.

It is safe to assume that the older patient may have several deficits that result from poor nutritional habits. Many older patients are in a state of semistarvation. Protein and vitamin deficits are common. Depletion of body protein leads to intracellular potassium loss with a resulting deficit of this ion. Potassium depletion in moderate amounts is believed to jeopardize the life of the aged surgical patient much more than is the case in younger patients.

A major emphasis in the preoperative nursing care of the elderly is attention to food and water intake. The diet is planned with the doctor and the dietitian. The diet should contain adequate amounts of protein. In order to encourage eating, the patient's likes and dislikes should be considered. Older patients often do better if they can be served frequent small meals. Enriched drinks may be well taken, and sufficient fluid should be given.

The elderly preoperative patient should be physically active, and ambulation is as important preoperatively as postoperatively. The preoperative period is the best time for the nurse to teach the patient the exercises he will be expected to do postoperatively.

In the postoperative period the patient is watched for signs of hypoxia, to which the elderly patient is particularly sensitive. Proper positioning to facilitate drainage of fluids from the respiratory tract is essential.

Most elderly patients receive water, electrolytes, and blood postoperatively. The rate of flow should be moderate in order not to present a too rapid increase of water and solute to the kidney for excretion. If fluid is administered too rapidly, with resultant expansion of the blood volume, there may be circulatory overloading leading to pulmonary edema. Water intoxication may be produced by the parenteral, subcutaneous, or rectal administration of water. If the patient can take fluids by mouth, tea, broth, diluted fruit juices, and water are given as soon as possible. Early return to a full diet is ideal. Once the patient is back on a satisfactory diet, every possible consideration should be given to his whims. A regular diet with an adequate amount of protein is essential for wound repair. A simple high-protein drink consists of 100 gm of skimmed-milk powder in a glass of milk.

Narcotics and sedatives should be used only as necessary and in the smallest dose that will achieve the desired result. Elderly patients are unusually sensitive to these drugs, and they may cause respiratory depression and consequent respiratory acidosis.

Early ambulation, deep breathing, turning, coughing, and bed exercises are essential in the postoperative care of the aged. They prevent atelectasis, pulmonary edema, embolus and thrombus formation, and abdominal distention. There are less nausea and vomiting. Early activity improves appetite, which leads to increased food intake. All these measures help to prevent or minimize fluid and electrolyte imbalances in the geriatric surgical patient and reduce the need for prolonged parenteral maintenance.

REFERENCE

1. SILVER, H.; KEMPE, C.; and BRUYN, H.: *Handbook of Pediatrics*. Large Medical Publishers, Los Altos, Calif., 1965.

ADDITIONAL READINGS

ARMSTRONG, I. L., and BROWDER, J. J.: *The Nursing Care of Children*. F. A. Davis, Philadelphia, 1964.

BELAND, I.: "Essentials of Geriatric Nursing" in Steiglitz, E. *Geriatric Medicine.* J. B. Lippincott, Philadelphia, 1954.

BRUSILOW, S., and COOKE, R.: "Fluid Therapy of Diarrhea and Vomiting," *Pediat Clin N Amer*, **6**:99, 1959.

CHOPE, H., and VRESLOW, K.: "Nutritional Status of the Aging," *J Public Health*, **46**:61, 1956.

FRIIS-HANSEN, B.: "Body Water Compartments in Children: Changes During Growth and Related Changes in Body Composition," *Pediat*, **28**:169, 1961.

HERRON, P.; JESSEPH, J.; and HARKINS, H.: "Analysis of 600 Operations in Patients over 70 Years of Age," *Ann Surg*, **152**:686, 1960.

MARLOW, D., and SELLEW, R.: *Textbook of Pediatric Nursing.* W. B. Saunders, Philadelphia, 1961.

NELSON, W.: *Textbook of Pediatrics.* W. B. Saunders, Philadelphia, 1960.

SHOCK, N.: "The Role of the Kidney in Electrolyte and Water Regulation in the Aged," *Ciba Foundation Colloquia on Ageing*, **4**:229, 1958.

STIEGLITZ, E.: *Geriatric Medicine.* J. B. Lippincott, Philadelphia, 1954.

Glossary

acid. A proton donor; substance that gives hydrogen (a proton) to another substance, rendering it more acid.

acidosis. A condition in which the total concentration of buffer base is reduced below normal, leaving a relatively greater concentration of hydrogen. A pH below 7.35.

agglutination. A phenomenon consisting of the collection into clumps of the cells distributed in a fluid; believed to be caused by molecules of agglutinins that become attached to the cells.

agglutinin. Antibody that aggregates a particular antigen, e.g., bacteria, following combination with homologous antigen.

agglutinogen. Any substance that, acting as an antigen, stimulates the production of agglutinin.

aldosterone. Hormone secreted by the adrenals that affects fluid and electrolyte balance.

alkali reserve. Term used to refer to the sodium in the blood that is in combination with bicarbonate. Called alkali reserve because the sodium can be used to combine with other anions.

alkaline solution. One in which the concentration of hydroxyl ions exceeds that of hydrogen ions.

alkalosis. A condition in which the total concentration of buffer base is greater than normal, with a relative decrease in hydrogen ion concentration; a pH higher than 7.45.

anabolism. Constructive metabolism; any constructive process by which simple substances are converted by living cells into more complex compounds.

anion. A particle that carries a negative charge in solution and will migrate to a positive pole (anode) if an electric current is passed through the solution, e.g., chloride, bicarbonate, phosphate, sulfate.

antigen. A substance, usually protein or protein-polysaccharide complex, that, when foreign to the blood, will stimulate formation of specific antibody if it gains entrance to the blood.

base. A proton acceptor; takes hydrogen (a proton) from a solution, rendering it less acid.

186

buffer. Substance that, by various chemical combinations, lessens the change in hydrogen ion concentration that otherwise would be produced by adding acids or alkalis.

buffer system. Pairs of chemicals in definite relationship to one another, which serve to maintain normal pH; the pairs consist of a weak acid and a salt formed by neutralizing the weak acid with a strong base; the weak acid, by releasing fewer hydrogen ions than the strong acid, serves to maintain pH.

calorie. A unit of heat.

calorie, large. Kilocalorie; the amount of heat necessary to raise the temperature of 1 kg of water 1°C; it is the unit used in the study of metabolism; abbreviated Cal.

calorie, small. The amount of heat required to raise the temperature of 1 gm of water 1°C; it is one thousandth of the large calorie; abbreviated cal.

catabolism. Destructive metabolism; the process involved in the conversion of body substances from complex to simple compounds.

cation. Particle that carries a positive charge in solution and will migrate to a negative pole (cathode) if an electric current is passed through the solution, e.g., sodium, hydrogen, potassium.

chloride shift. A buffering activity in which a chloride ion leaves an erythrocyte for each bicarbonate ion entering it, or in which a chloride ion enters an erythrocyte for each bicarbonate ion leaving it, in an attempt to maintain electroneutrality.

colloid osmotic pressure. Pressure that results from dispersed colloid particles.

contraction-of-fluid phase. Decrease in fluid volume; dehydration.

cut-down. Surgical incision to expose a vein for venoclysis.

dehydration. Decrease in fluid volume; contraction-of-fluid phase.

dependent edema. Increase in fluid volume in areas in which gravity and position are determining factors, e.g., the ankles in the standing position.

diffusion. Movement of particles from the area of their highest concentration to the area of their least concentration; an attempt to maintain balance between anions and cations.

edema. Increase in fluid volume in any fluid space; most frequently seen in interstitial space; expansion-of-fluid phase.

electrolyte. Substance that dissociates into ions in solution and carries an electric charge.

enteral. Within the alimentary tract.

equivalent. The unit of measurement of chemical activity of a substance; the number of grams of an element that will combine with 8 gm of oxygen or 1.008 gm of hydrogen; the sum of atomic weights of an ion divided by its valence.

eschar. The dehydrated, dead skin produced by burning; slough.

fixed cation or anion. That which is not destroyed in metabolism and which must be excreted by the kidney.

fluid phase. Term used to designate the man-designated fluid compartments in the body.

hemolysis.   Separation of the hemoglobin from the corpuscles and appearance of the hemoglobin in the fluid in which the corpuscles are suspended.

homeostasis.   Term meaning dynamic equilibrium within the body.

hydrostatic pressure.   The force exerted by a fluid against the wall of the chamber in which it is contained.

hyperkalemia.   An increase in serum potassium.

hypernatremia.   An increase in serum sodium.

hypertonic.   Having a greater amount of solute or a higher osmotic pressure than solution to which it is compared.

hypodermoclysis.   Subcutaneous feeding.

hypokalemia.   A decrease in serum potassium.

hyponatremia.   A decrease in serum sodium.

hypotonic.   Having a smaller amount of solute or less osmotic pressure than solution to which it is compared.

iatrogenic.   Induced by the physician; resulting from the activity of the physician or from treatment.

infiltration.   The accumulation in a tissue of substances not normal to it; seen when fluid seeps out of the vascular space into the interstitial space.

insensible water loss.   That which is lost without awareness of the person, e.g., through the lungs or stool.

interstitial.   Outside of the cells within the tissue spaces.

intracellular.   Within the cell.

intravascular.   Within the blood vessel; the plasma.

ion.   An atom that carries an electric charge in solution.

ionization.   Process of dissociation of electrolytes in solution.

iso-osmotic.   Isotonic; having the same amount of solute or osmotic pressure as substance to which it is compared.

isotonic.   Having the same amount of solute or osmotic pressure as substance to which it is compared.

ketosis.   The accumulation in the body of ketone bodies: acetone, beta-hydroxybutyric acid, aceto-acetic acid.

kilogram.   1000 gm.

metabolism.   The sum of all the physical and chemical processes by which living organized substance is produced and maintained and through which energy is made available for use.

milliequivalent.   The unit of measurement of chemical activity; 1/1000 of an equivalent (see equivalent).

milliequivalent per liter. $\dfrac{mg/100\ ml \times 10 \times valence}{atomic\ weight}$.

millimol.   1/1000 of a mol; (see mol).

milliosmol.   1/1000 of an osmol; indicates the osmotic activity of separate ions of an electrolyte (see milliosmol per liter).

milliosmol per liter. $\dfrac{mg/100\ ml \times 10}{atomic\ weight}$.

mol.   Molecular weight of a substance in grams.

molal solution. One containing 1 gm molecular weight of solute in 1 kg of solution; moles per 1000 gm.

molar solution. One containing 1 gm molecular weight of solute in each liter of solution; moles per 1000 ml.

negative nitrogen balance. Loss of greater amounts of nitrogen than are replaced; decreased protein intake.

obligatory water loss. Water lost by vaporization from lungs and skin and in feces, which goes on even when environmental temperatures are low.

oncotic pressure. Colloid osmotic pressure; pressure that results from dispersed colloid particles.

osmolality. Term used to indicate the number of particles in a given space or the gram molecular weight in kilograms of solution; osmolality of plasma is 290 mOs; used when studying physical properties of both solute and solvent, e.g., freezing points.

osmolarity. Term used to indicate the gram molecular weight of solute in each liter of solution; used in volume analyses to determine concentration of solutes.

osmosis. Passage of solvent through a semipermeable membrane from an area of lesser concentration of solute to an area of greater concentration of solute.

osmotic pressure. Pressure caused by continuous movement of concentration of molecules; the greater the number of molecules, the greater the osmotic pressure.

parenteral. Outside the alimentary tract.

pH. Simplified expression of hydrogen ion concentration and/or activity or acidity; equals the negative logarithm of the hydrogen ion concentration.

pK. Negative logarithm of dissociation constant of buffers; mathematically determined ionization possibility of a buffer; determined by measuring the pH of a solution that contains equal concentrations of the two components that make up a buffer pair.

refractory edema. Expansion of fluid phase, which is not improved following adequate therapeutic regimen.

sensible water loss. Water loss that can be seen and felt, over and above insensible loss.

thin-wall needle. Needle that has an inside diameter one size larger than its gauge.

titer. The quantity of a substance required to produce a reaction with a given volume of another substance; the highest dilution of a serum that causes clumping of bacteria.

unfixed cation or anion. Those that are disposed of as carbon dioxide and water and do not require activity by the kidney.

venoclysis. Intravenous feeding.

Index

Acid, definition, 31
  nonvolatile, 39
  renal excretion, 39
  volatile, 39
Acid-base regulation, 30–39
  renal influences, 38–39
  respiratory influences, 37–38
Acidemia, 44
Acidifying salts, as diuretics, 76
Acidifying solutions, 162
Acidosis, 43–54
  clinical signs, 48–50
  compensatory devices, 43–45
  complications of therapy, 59–60
  laboratory studies, 45–47
  metabolic, 47–52
    carbohydrate and protein metabolism, 47
    compensatory devices, 48
    in the geriatric patient, 182
    a patient care study, 48–52
  nursing care, 57–60
  replacement solutions, 163
  respiratory, 52–54
    compensatory devices, 52–53
  treatment, 50–52
Adrenal glands, in water and salt imbalance, 64–65
Agglutination, in transfusion reactions, 166
Air embolus, from blood transfusion, 168
Albumin-globulin ratio, 45
Alcohol, nursing during administration of, 171–74
  in replacement therapy, 158

and suppression of antidiuretic hormone, 66
  table of solutions, 158
Aldactone, 76, 93
Aldosterone, 16, 22, 65, 91–92
  in congenital heart failure, 77
  in water and electrolyte imbalance, 64
Aldosteronism, primary, 92
  secondary, 92
Alkalemia, 44
Alkalosis, 54–57
  compensatory devices, 43–45
  complications of therapy, 59–60
  laboratory studies, 45–47
  metabolic, 54–56
  milk-alkali syndrome, 55
  nursing care, 57–60
  respiratory, 56–57
  treatment, 54–56
Ammonia, 47
Ammonium chloride, as diuretic, 76
  in gastric replacement solution, 163
  parenteral solution, 162
  in treatment of metabolic acidosis, 56, 60
Anesthesia, degree of, in burns, 126
  metabolic acidosis, 48
Anion, 5
  and cations, table of, in normal serum or plasma, 180
Antacids, metabolic alkalosis, 56
Anticoagulant-preservative for blood collection, 172
Antidiuretic hormone, 15–16
  in diabetes insipidus, 67

Antidiuretic hormone [*Cont.*]
  production of, after surgery, 66
  in water and salt imbalance, 64,
    65, 72
Antigens, in blood groups, 165–66
Aqueous silver nitrate, for burns, 134
Artificial kidney, in potassium
    toxicity, 105
Ascites, paracentesis for, 83
Aspirin and salicylate poisoning, a
    patient study, 178–81
Autografts, in burn treatment, 139

Base, definition, 31
Basilic vein, for intravenous
    administration, 152
Bicarbonate ion, in acidosis and
    alkalosis, 43–45, 48, 56, 57
  in multielectrolyte solutions, 163
  in salicylate poisoning, 179
Blood, administration, 172–74
  collection, with anticoagulant
    preservative, 172
  cross matching and typing, 166, 167,
    172
  factors, 167
  groups, 164–66
  recipient and donor, 166
  storage, 172
Blood infusion, 167–70
  complications, 168–70
  nursing responsibilities, 172–74
  Rh incompatibility, 169
Blood pressure, leg reading, 136–37
Blood serum, chemistry (table), 46
  normal ranges of cations and anions, 19
Blood urea nitrogen values, 45
Body buffers in blood, 34–35
Body liquids, functions, 5
Body surface area nomogram, 143–44
Bone, and the extracellular fluid, 23–24
Breathing exercises, for geriatric
    patients, 181
Brooke Army Medical Center formula,
    in treatment of burns, 134
Buffer pairs in blood, 35
Buffer mechanisms in respiratory
    alkalosis, 57

Buffer systems, 34
  in blood, 35
Buffering, in pH control, 44
Buffering action, definition, 34
Burns, 125–39
  crust formation, 127
  depth, 128
  diuresis, 135–36
  hypovolemia, 132
  inflammatory response, 132
  nursing care, 136, 139
    positioning, 138
    record of intake and output, 137–38
  a patient care study, 125–28
  percentage of body involvement, 126,
    128, 129, 132
  phases, 133–36
  postshock phase, 135–36
  shock, 133–34
  treatment, debridement, 136
    diet, 135–36, 138–39
    intravenous therapy, 137–38
    pHisoHex treatment, 127, 138
    physical therapy, 138–39
    tetanus antitoxin, 126
    use of autografts, 139
    use of ice water, 127
    wet dressings, 138
  weight gain, 136
Burn shock, use of saline, 133, 135
Burn team, 126
Butler's solution, 163

Calcitonin, 119
Calcium, 22–24, 118
  in blood serum, 46
  deficit of, 120. *See also* Hypocalcemia
  excess of, 120
  gluconate, for hypocalcemia, 52, 59, 60
  solutions and blood, 173
  in urine, 47
Calculators, for determining intravenous
    drops per minute, 150
Calories in parenteral solutions,
    157–58
Capillary membrane and edema, 74
Carbohydrate, requirements per
    square meter of body surface
    area, 144